Dementia]
Everyday Mini-Miracles
Through Food, Vitamins and Supplements©

Forward by: Dr. Mordy Levy, MD, DC, ND
By Shari Darling

http://www.dementiadiet.net

For additional information please contact:

http://www.dementiadiet.net

or at shariLdarling@gmail.com

Special Thanks to My Editors

Dr. Mordy Levy

Deanna Shanti, Shanti Publishing

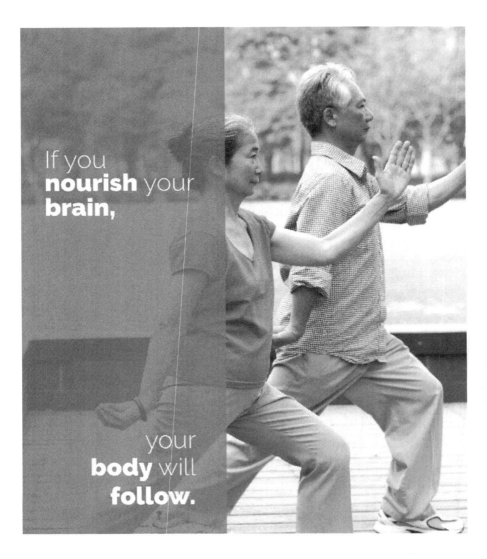
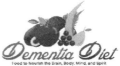

Acknowledgement:

I acknowledge my husband, Jack, for his graciousness, generosity of spirit, incredible ability to love and forgive, his courage, wisdom and magnificence. Jack is a man of great integrity. He is an extraordinary husband, ex-husband and father of five incredible children who are a contribution to the human race.

I realized the depth of my husband's courage on the day Dr. Finlayson, his neurologist, diagnosed Jack with Alzheimer's. We left the doc's office and went to a restaurant for an early dinner. We were quiet. Sitting across from Jack I looked into his eyes. I could not read what he was thinking. I was scared. Shocked. I finally muttered, "So what do you think of this diagnosis?"

In that quiet and assured Navy SEAL Commander (Ret.) confidence, he replied,

> *"You really don't know who you are until you take on something much greater than yourself."*

I felt the tears running down my cheeks. Like a Navy SEAL ready for a mission on the spur of a moment, Jack was, in that moment, ready to take on what some might say the greatest war of his life.

Learning of his diagnosis of Alzheimer's was devastating. However, I also feel blessed to be able to spend more of our lives together. I have a friend who lost his wife suddenly and unexpectedly. This, for me, is far worse. Jack's Alzheimer's has given us a new life perspective. We have stopped racing through our days. I have become far more patient and compassionate toward Jack. We have both started to enjoy each day, each moment, moment by moment with each other and those we love. You know you are living in the moment when you experience peace.

I also acknowledge our functional medicine physician, Dr. Mordy Levy, MD, DC, ND

He is my other Mr. Right! Without Dr. Levy's extensive testing and vitamin and supplement regime for Jack, I don't know where Jack would be today with respect to his Alzheimer's symptoms. Dr. Levy is a brilliant, passionate and compassionate medical physician, as well as a naturopathic doctor and chiropractor. He treats the whole human being in all of its intricate facets and details. Dr. Levy is a God-send to us. Thank you Dr. Levy.

Dementia Diet: Everyday Mini-Miracles -- Through diet, vitamins and supplements

Table of Contents

Forward: By Dr. Mordy Levy, MD, DC, ND

"I dedicate this forward in the memory of my dear grandmother Hannah, who passed away from Alzheimer's disease."

- Dr. Mordy Levy

Dementia Diet: Everyday Mini-Miracles is a unique compilation of numerous dietary interventions for dementia. It shares the story of one of my patients, Jack, who struggles with dementia, and his caregiver, Shari, who continues to do a fantastic job researching the disease, finding numerous evidence-based natural alternative remedies, from special diets and supplements to lifestyle changes.

Although the emphasis of this extensive work is on dementia, specifically Alzheimer disease, the unique individualized approach of functional medicine is for all chronic diseases. Functional medicine addresses the person instead of the disease. It connects the dots among all organ-based systems. It restores impaired mechanisms to proper function. This is opposite of the existing paradigm of traditional medicine focusing on specific diseases.

Alzheimer disease is one of many chronic and debilitating diseases that can be systematically helped with functional medicine. I would encourage you to be proactive with your health, to seek an integrative and functional medicine doctor. These are doctors who are trained to think differently. Doctors who will take the time to listen to their patients' stories. Doctors who will apply their medical knowledge and investigate for the root of the problem, instead of prescribing drugs for key symptoms.

As a doctor, I witnessed many "miracles" or as what some physicians label "spontaneous remissions" due to the systematic therapeutic approach of functional medicine. Chronic fatigue patients gain back their youthful energy. Insomniacs finally enjoy restful sleep. Asthmatics gain new understanding to the meaning of "breath of fresh air". Individuals with severe atopic dermatitis no longer need to hide behind layers of clothes and a mask of makeup. Parkinson's patients who can finally sign their names, and Alzheimer's patients who have a return of lost memories.

Functional Medicine is a paradigm shift in the way we think about health, disease, and medicine. Together we can help shape the future of healthcare and achieve the ultimate universal goal of disease prevention and health promotion.

Sincerely,

Mordy Levy, MD, DC, ND
Practice in Integrative and Functional Medicine
http://www.DrLevy.ca
Toronto, Ontario, Canada

Preface: Dementia

Every four seconds across the planet a new case of dementia is diagnosed.

In 2010 about 35.6 million people worldwide were living with dementia. This statistic will double by 2030 and triple by 2050. There are likely as many caregivers on the planet – 35.6 million – who are caring for a loved one with dementia. About 58% of this number live in low to middle-income countries, and this proportion is projected to rise to 71% by 2050.

In North America, Alzheimer's is at epidemic proportions. One in eight people over the age of sixty-five live with this disease.

Global costs of dementia on health care systems is astronomical.

In the United States, alone, the cost of dementia on the health care system is $604 billion per year.

Dementia devastates families. Stresses include physical, emotional and economic pressures. Caregivers require support from their community and their country's health, social, financial and legal systems. In the United States more than fifteen million Americans provide more than seventeen billion hours each year of unpaid care to loved ones with Alzheimer's. (Alzheimer's Association).

Early diagnosis will improve the quality of life of people with dementia, as well as for their caregivers and families.

We don't have all the answers yet, but there is overwhelming and growing evidence that regular intake of certain foods, nutrients and supplements can help keep your brain healthy and reduce your risk of developing dementia. Jack and I can claim, through first-hand experience, that food, nutrients and supplements have nourished his malnourished brain, thus reversing some of the cognitive and bodily symptoms. By reversing symptoms we are, in essence, slowing the progression of his dementia, giving him quality of life for a longer time and returning him back to himself for as long as possible.

Several nutrients and particular diets have been linked to maintaining healthy brain cells and reducing the risk of dementia. "Dementia Diet: Everyday Mini-Miracles" is the name of this book. However "Dementia Diet©" is also the name of our series of books dealing with all aspects of dementia and life for both the caregivers and the person with dementia. The series includes books that will educate on foods and supplements that nourish the body and brain, as well as food for thought to nourish the mind and spirit. We live in the possibility of slowing the progression of dementia for all those who suffer from this disease. One day perhaps there will be a cure.

This Book:

"A miracle is a shift in perspective.

-- Cora Whittington

In the Merriam-Webster dictionary, a miracle has several meanings, including 'an extremely outstanding or unusual event, thing, or accomplishment.' The word 'miracle' is described in dictionary.com as a wonder and marvel.

I chose the title 'Everyday Mini-Miracles' because that is what I've witnessed. Mini-miracles in Jack's everyday functions -- the small but important returns to himself in mind, body and spirit -- as outstanding and marvellous. I like the word 'return to oneself 'or just 'return' rather than the word 'improvement(s)'. One cannot improve with dementia. But some of the symptoms of dementia can be subsided and reversed so that the person returns back to being him/herself.

I also like the word 'miracle' because it offers hope in the face of an existing dark and scientific paradigm where most experts say there is no known means for slowing the progression and no cure for Alzheimer's and other types of dementia. It is when a caregiver and a person with dementia buy into this perspective

4

that life becomes hard and hopeless and resignation and depression set in.

This need not be the case. In the face of Jack's dementia we have lost the lust, but gained more romance. We have grown closer – emotionally and spiritually. We are taking this journey together. On some days Jack might feel frustrated; I get impatient. But the feelings come and go. As Jack says, "Feelings do nothing more than tell you how you feel. They don't make a difference." Maybe that's a SEAL mantra, one he used to tell himself when undergoing extreme adversities in BUD/s training or when in combat. (He served three tours in Vietnam).

Most of the time we are at peace with this journey and look for opportunities to make a difference in our own wellbeing and in the lives of others. I can say that I experience for Jack a greater depth of love and respect today than I have ever have.

I wrote this book for many reasons. Bringing awareness and understanding of dementia across all levels of society and community is needed to improve the quality of life for persons with dementia and the quality of life for their caregivers and families.

Dementia should be a concern for everyone because it is an epidemic that will continue to severely tax our health care systems.

I also wanted to share with you the wonderful everyday mini-miracles that Jack has experienced through his diet, vitamins and supplements to give you hope that you too can do the same. Only caregivers understand the joy and relief we experience when the person with dementia, the person we love so deeply, shows signs of tangible returning to oneself in mind, body and/or spirit.

In this book I share with you the dietary lifestyle that we researched, created and implemented into Jack's life as well as my own.

This is not a scientific or medical study on dementia. I possess no medical background of any kind. I am, however, an investigative journalist by trade. Through the knowledge I've gained through research and from Dr. Levy, I bring to you our own personal perspectives and journey and proof.

While dementia may be a life sentence, it doesn't mean one must give up on life.

Our hope is that this book will provide you with gems of information that will make a difference for you in your life. We hope the information will make a difference and bring about health, whether you have dementia or you are a caregiver like me.

If you acquire only one piece of information that inspires you to action to improve your health or supports you in improving quality of life for you and your loved one, Jack and I will have done our job.

I stress that you first consult your physician before implementing any new dietary plan or adding any new vitamins and supplements to your dietary plan.

Chapter 1: Introduction:

You, the Reader:

Throughout this book I refer to you, the reader. You may be a caregiver like me. Or you may be someone pre-disposed to dementia or in the early to moderate stages of living with this disease. From whatever perspective you come, I address you directly. I acknowledge you for being open-minded and for standing in the possibility of improving quality of life for yourself.

The Chapters:

The chapters cover the Dementia Diet principles in more detail.

The principles are meant to improve the health of the brain, body, mind and spirit and quality of life for everyone – the person with dementia, as well as caregivers and family members.

At the end of each chapter you'll find a section called "In an organic nutshell." This section is for you if you simply need to know the information, the main points, without an explanation. Scroll down to this section. You will be provided with the key points of each chapter.

Definition of Dementia:

Many people use the term dementia as though it is a single disease. It is not. Or they diagnose Alzheimer's for those with other forms of dementia. Dementia is a general term to describe an umbrella or collection of wide-range signs and symptoms resulting from illnesses, disease or trauma to the brain. It is the loss of cognitive functioning, eventually severe enough to impact and reduce a person's ability to think, remember, reason, and to speak. It also can impact a person's behavior and bodily functions.

Dementia can be reversible, such as is the case with thyroid problems or vitamin deficiencies or in the case of abstaining from alcohol. There is actually alcohol induced dementia. It can also be static, such as from brain injury. Or dementia can be progressive with long-term decline due to damage or disease of the brain (as is the case with Alzheimer's, Lewy Body and vascular dementia).

Dementia is also often incorrectly called 'senility' or 'senile dementia' because it primarily affects older people. Senility is the state of being senile, especially with old age. Dementia is a chronic or progressive syndrome of serious mental decline, which is not a normal part of aging. They are not the same.

Types of Dementia:

The primary types of dementia are as follows:

- Alzheimer's Disease
- Vascular Dementia (occurs after a stroke)
- Mixed Dementia
- Frontotemporal
- Lewy Body Dementia
- Huntington Disease
- Parkinson Disease Dementia
- Pick Disease
- Cruetzfeld-Jakob Disease

Research:

In over fifty years of living I've discovered that there is never only one answer or one truth or one miracle cure or remedy for any ailment. Especially when it comes to disease. As mentioned in the preface, Jack's healthy body and positive state of being, in the face of this disease in its moderate stage, is due to a combination of factors.

There are endless ways to pursue one's life and one's health. The art is in finding the right path for you and in this case, perhaps the right health path for your loved one living with some form of dementia. It must also be a path that is closely monitored by a trusted physician.

There is plenty of research for and against every ingredient we eat. This book does not aim to use in-depth scientific studies to validate any point of view. I am sharing our personal viewpoint, our journey, based on the information we've discovered. And more importantly how this information fits into our own beliefs and lifestyle.

Here are four of the food diets believed to be beneficial for persons with dementia:

Paleo Diet:

The Paleo Diet suggests that refined foods, trans fats and sugar are at the heart of degenerative diseases, such as Alzheimer's, Parkinson's, diabetes, heart disease, depression and infertility. On this diet one consumes lean proteins, fruits and vegetables, seafood, nuts and seeds and healthy fats. It advocates that dairy, grains, processed food and sugars, legumes, starches and alcohol should be avoided.

Grain Brain Approach:

Through research I discovered a book called 'Grain Brain: The Surprising Truth About Wheat, Carbs, and Sugar – Your Brain's Silent Killers,' written by David Perlmutter. Dr. Perlmutter is a renowned and board-certified neurologist and a fellow of the American College of Nutrition. I highly recommend this book. Dr. Perlmutter advocates a fat-rich, low-carbohydrate diet. He believes carbohydrates are destroying our brains – even the ones that are touted as healthy like whole grains. This Florida-based neurologist believes that carbs can cause dementia, ADHD, anxiety, chronic headaches, depression, and much more.

In his book Dr. Perlmutter explains what happens when the brain encounters a daily consumption of breads and pastas, grains and even some fruit and why our brains actually thrive on fats and cholesterol. And more importantly, Dr. Perlmutter states that we can spur the growth of new brain cells at any age.

In Grain Brain, he offers an in-depth look at how we can take control of our "smart genes" through specific dietary choices and lifestyle habits, demonstrating how to remedy our most feared maladies without drugs.

The Alzheimer's Association Diet Recommendation:

The Alzheimer's Association believes the brain requires a diet that is low in fat and cholesterol, is balanced in nutrients and includes protein and sugar.

The ALZ (www.alz.org) states on its website, "According to the most current research, a brain-healthy diet is one that reduces the risk of heart disease and diabetes, encourages good blood flow to the brain, and is low in fat and cholesterol. Like the heart, the brain needs the right balance of nutrients, including protein and sugar, to function well. A brain-healthy diet is most effective when combined with physical and mental activity and social interaction."

Mayo Clinic Approach:

I also found that the Mayo Clinic offered yet a slightly different nutritional approach.

In a published article on (www.mayoclinic.org) entitled *Can a Mediterranean diet lower my risk of Alzheimer's?* Dr. Smith states, "You may know that a Mediterranean diet — rich in fruits, vegetables, olive oil, legumes, whole grains and fish — offers heart-healthy benefits. But a Mediterranean diet may also benefit your brain. Studies show that people who closely follow a Mediterranean diet seem less likely to develop cognitive decline when compared with people who don't follow the diet."

10

Research shows that a Mediterranean diet may:

"Reduce the risk of mild cognitive impairment, a transitional stage between the cognitive decline of normal aging and the more-serious memory problems caused by dementia or Alzheimer's disease...It's unclear why following a Mediterranean diet may protect brain function. Researchers speculate that making healthy food choices may improve cholesterol and blood sugar levels and overall blood vessel health — all factors that may reduce the risk of mild cognitive impairment or Alzheimer's disease....More research is needed to know to what degree a Mediterranean diet prevents Alzheimer's or slows the progression of cognitive decline. Nonetheless, eating a healthy diet is important to stay physically and mentally fit."

Our Approach:

All these diets are believed to be beneficial. For Jack and I, however, they seemed somewhat unrealistic in one way or another to maintain on a day-to-day basis, as well as month to month and year after year. I'm not making the diets wrong. They are all legitimate, scientifically approven approaches to a healthy lifestyle. However, we required a more individualized diet that we knew we could both maintain on a long-term basis. Again, there is no cookie-cutter answer to handling the dietary needs of a person with dementia or the caregiver. Every person has his/her own dietary requirements.

It takes a team to combat dementia. Dr. Levy is our medical expert. As a caregiver I cook the food and set up the system for Jack to take his vitamins and supplements daily. Jack is highly coachable and implements whatever is given to him. We share with you our journey and discoveries.

Chapter 2: Jack and The Dementia Diet©

Jack:

Jack is twenty-one years older than I. At age seventy-four he was finally diagnosed with Alzheimer's disease. I say 'finally' because I knew on some level, instinctively, for seven years before this diagnosis that he was suffering from some form of dementia. Our local memory clinic failed to identify it, despite my constant concern and communication with them. As any caregiver will share, the journey to diagnosis is discombobulating, enraging, heart breaking, and frustrating.

In his mid-sixties, Jack began to show signs of short-term memory decline. He could not recall a telephone conversation moments after he hung up. He also had difficulty locating objects sitting directly in front of him. I thought it was a bad habit and summed it up to laziness. Sometimes, when dining with friends he would snap at me unexpectedly and then be oblivious to how embarrassed I felt.

I also noticed significant changes and decline in Jack's functions and cognitive skills after his hip replacement surgery and carotid artery surgery and while having to take medications for blood thinning, high cholesterol and blood pressure.

It became my personal agenda to understand his progressing cognitive decline. I was scared. His anger episodes subsided, replaced by calm and overall confusion. Jack was highly intelligent and an avid reader. 'Avid' is understated. He could demolish an entire book in one sitting or within a day, even a thick one. After retirement and with a love of reading Jack went from reading an average of fifteen to twenty books per month to not being able to read even one, not able to understand a single sentence. He said reading was no longer enjoyable because he could not retain the meaning of the words and had to keep re-reading the first sentence of the first chapter.

No longer could he understand basic movie plots. His childhood memories became a focus. When I would change the subject, Jack would listen and then go right back to where he left off in his childhood story. A story I had heard countless times. For many years during tax season Jack would balance my finances down to the penny. After the surgeries, Jack struggled with using a calculator.

He began to talk to himself while wide-awake and he experienced waking hallucinations.

Upon my request, Jack's doctor referred him to a clinic that deals, among many things, with memory. At this medical clinic Jack underwent a series of tests. It seemed that the medical assistants who performed the tests helped Jack with the answers. I would say, "Are you supposed to be helping him?" They just ignored my question.

A general practitioner, not someone who specialized in dementia, saw Jack. This physician told us that Jack had had a stroke leaving cognitive impairment. The physician said his cognitive ability had declined but was stable.

But Jack was not stable. He continued to decline. His symptoms worsened. I kept calling the clinic requesting they see Jack again. They said that it could 'appear' that he was declining if he was stressed out. And we were undergoing a great deal of stress at that time. I begged for another test. They tested him twice and in both cases the physician stated that Jack's cognition was stable.

I knew different. I could see the decline taking hold. Knowing the truth and having a doctor tell you otherwise is frustrating and agonizing. I knew I was not imagining the decline.

I finally poured my heart out to Jack's cardiologist. The cardiologist noticed that Jack did not understand what was being told to him about his heart, that he had arterial fibrillation. The cardiologist immediately referred Jack to a neurologist.

The neurologist tested Jack and afterwards shared her findings. She believed Jack might have Lewy Body Dementia (LBD) due to one particular kind of hallucination of a woman and the severe muscle cramping in his legs. She said it might also be Parkinson's Dementia Disease. The neurologist ordered a CAT scan and an MRI. I moved through the shock, grief and sadness. After undergoing further testing and in interpreting the CAT and MRI, the neurologist told us that Jack had never had a stroke at all. She diagnosed him with Alzheimer's disease.

This diagnosis was devastating, but also gave me a sense of where we needed to start, a sense of clarity and direction. We were finally getting the right help.

The neurologist prescribed a drug called Exelon. Exelon (rivastigmine) improves the function of nerve cells in the brain. It works by preventing the breakdown of a chemical that is important for the processes of memory, thinking, and reasoning. People with dementia usually have lower levels of this chemical, I was told.

Exelon is used to treat mild to moderate dementia caused by Alzheimer's or Parkinson's disease. (Take note that I am not advocating Exelon for all dementia patients. I am simply sharing our personal story).

Exelon gave Jack more clarity of mind. The cloud of complete fog seemed to disappear. Over time I noticed that he had stopped mentally declining. He was not getting worse. But Jack still dealt with many cognitive and physical 'dys-functions' that had already taken hold.

I refused to believe that this was as good as it was going to get. I am of the belief that we don't get as much nutrition as we should from the foods we eat. So I wondered if some of Jack's symptoms could be from a lack of nutrition as opposed to being due to dementia. Hence, I started on a journey to complement this allopathic approach with a nutrition-based, naturopathic one.

14

The Dementia Diet:

It is through research, being monitored and coached by doctors, altering our own diet and lifestyle and experiencing the returns to health of Jack's brain, body, mind, and spirit (as well as my own) that we were inspired to develop the Dementia Diet.

At the moment there is no definitive treatment for dementia. Allopathic medicine concludes that there is no cognitive cure for the brain. Through the use of MRI and CAT scans only his neurologist can state that Jack's brain has experienced change.

We can attest that the Dementia Diet is healing Jack's brain, body, mind and spirit. You might ask, "Spirit?" Yes, Jack's spirit. When we become physically healthy, our life, attitude, perspectives and mood improves, thus positively affecting our spirit.

The Dementia Diet is also a healthy lifestyle approach for everyone, not just for those with dementia or Alzheimer's. This philosophy will nourish the brain, body, mind and spirit of caregivers, too. And this is just as important.

The emotional and physical strain that comes from caring for a loved one with Alzheimer's or dementia is enormous. On average caregiving responsibilities can last from 10 to 15 years. During this time, caregivers experience health issues, such as physical illnesses and problems, along with depression, anxiety and substance abuse. Research now shows that Alzheimer's caregivers have a 63% higher mortality rate than non-caregivers. In fact 40% of Alzheimer's caregivers die from stress-related issues before their patients.

Everyone can return to a state of good health by following this lifestyle plan.

Alzheimer's Disease:

The cause of Alzheimer's disease is still not fully understood. What we know to date is that the Alzheimer's brain has fewer healthy cells and fewer connections between living cells than does a normal brain. As cells die, the brain shrinks. The brain develops two distinct abnormalities called plaques and tangles, now considered hallmarks of this particular form of dementia.

However, through much research and now validation by worldwide medical experts, another hallmark of this disease has been identified. It is called brain starvation or type 3 diabetes of the brain.

In the case of Alzheimer's, the Dementia Diet addresses brain starvation, as well as brain and body inflammation. The Dementia Diet has returned Jack from moderate-on-the-edge-of severe Alzheimer's to moderate and stable. Through our own personal journey and results I can confidently state that the Dementia Diet has aided in nourishing Jack's starved brain and has significantly reduced his brain and body inflammation!

So what exactly is brain starvation?

The Hallmarks of Alzheimer's:

First, allow me to provide a very brief, layman and simplistic explanation of this complicated disease called Alzheimer's.

Simply said, here are the hallmarks to the Alzheimer's brain. They are plaques, tangles, loss of connection, brain starvation, and inflammation.

Plaques: These clusters of protein fragments called beta-amyloid build up between nerve cells and destroy the brain by interfering with cell-to-cell communication.

16

Tangles: A healthy brain requires the normal structure and functioning of a protein called tau to transport nutrients and other essential materials throughout their long extensions. In the Alzheimer's brain, threads of tau protein twist into abnormal tangles inside brain cells. This leads to the failing of the transport system. As a result nutrients and these other essential materials cannot be transported throughout, thus causing brain cells to die.

Loss of Connection Between Brain Cells: Evidence suggests there is a loss of connection between brain cells that are responsible for memory, learning and communication. In the normal brain these connections (synapses) transmit information from cell to cell.

Brain Starvation: We all use sugar to provide energy to all the cells in our body. In the Alzheimer's brain there exists a problem with the glucose receptors and as a result the brain is slowly starved of glucose. A brain can be starved of glucose from 10 to even 30 years before signs of dementia are evident. This is believed to cause tissue shrinkable.

Inflammation: Inflammation is triggered by the body's immune system.

The Dementia Diet addresses the hallmarks of brain starvation and inflammation. The diet incorporates foods, vitamins and supplements that nourish the starved brain. This plan also suggests the elimination of specific foods to reduce brain and body inflammation, all of which is explained in more detail later on.

Our Personal Proof:

Pat Bolger is a long-time friend, a two-time Olympian, and physical education professor. At age sixty and at 5 feet and 6 inches he has a body fat content of about 15%. Pat taught me one of the greatest fitness lessons of my life. He said that people should simply take on the principles of discipline and consistency both at the dinner table and in exercising. This leads to a healthy body and a healthy weight, he said.

Taking Pat's lesson into life, the Dementia Diet is not a quick fix or fad diet based on setting seven day, thirty day or even 365-day goals. It's not a miracle cure. It is a holistic and practical approach to living to improve one's quality of life. Our goal is, of course, to slow the progression of Jack's dementia, but that can never really be measured or proven. It exists in both my and Jack's personal experience only.

Also note that you and your physician need to find out what works for you and tailor your diet to your specific health goals, food allergies, likes and dislikes. I advocate that you take in this information and use what you can to create your own health plan. Your health plan should be as individualistic as your fingerprint!

Sacrifice and starvation are also not part of this philosophy. One is not expected to count calories or points. This disease called dementia, and in my husband's case Alzheimer's, is already robbing Jack of elements of his quality of life. The last thing I want to do is remove even more of the things he loves, particularly the foods he loves. By the same token, there are ways to create healthy versions of the foods he loves, even ice cream! (Try our recipe for my Low Glycemic, Gluten-Free, Sugar Free, Dairy Free Starbucks Mocha Almond Ice Cream found in the book called *Dementia Diet: Everyday Mini-Miracles Cookbook*). Dementia Diet: Everyday Mini-Miracles Cookbook is available through Amazon.

Losing weight is also not a primary aim of this diet. The reason is that every person with dementia experiences his or her own weight challenges. Some people with dementia gain weight while others lose weight through loss of appetite. Brain health is the ultimate goal.

However, weight loss may be a natural benefit (if desired). Jack, for example, naturally moved from 230 pounds to 181 pounds within a year by incorporating the Dementia Diet into his life. He bares a healthy appetite, eating three meals per day and sometimes snacks in between. Jack feels better and looks better and has more energy.

Jack also has atrial fibrillation, an irregular and often rapid heart rate that commonly causes poor blood flow to the body. During atrial fibrillation, the heart's two upper chambers (the atria) beat chaotically and irregularly — out of coordination with the two lower chambers (the ventricles) of the heart. To prevent atrial fibrillation, some risk factors may be controlled or modified. These include high cholesterol, high blood pressure, heart disease, smoking, excess weight, caffeine, alcohol abuse, lack of exercise, some medications and sleep apnea.

Through the Dementia Diet Jack has eliminated these risk factors.

Due to his weight loss Jack has stopped snoring and holding his breath at night, thus is sleeping more soundly. He no longer requires the sleep apnea machine. Better quality of sleep has added to his clarity of mind and high energy level.

I can confidently state that through the Dementia Diet we have experienced a change in Jack's mind, body and spirit. This is due to a combination of elements. They are as follows:

- the Alzheimer's medication
- by incorporating a daily and individualized whole food vitamin and supplement regime designed by Dr. Levy.
- through improved sleep patterns due to weight loss
- through improved and increased regular exercise
- through the elimination of cigars
- limiting his wine consumption to a quarter of a glass every few weeks

- through the reduction of caffeine to one cappuccino per day
- by being active in our community and making a difference for others
- by incorporating the 7 Dementia Diet Principles (stated below)

7 Dementia Diet Principles:

As stated, the Dementia Diet focuses on nourishing the brain (and in the case of Alzheimer's, the starved brain) and suggests the elimination of foods to reduce brain and body inflammation.

The 7 Dementia Diet Principles are as follows:

1. Supplementing one's diet with a physician monitored vitamin/supplement regime.
2. Drastically lowering carbohydrate and sugar intake both natural and refined.
3. Being gluten and wheat-free.
4. Balancing one's diet with low glycemic fruits, vegetables and grains.
5. Eliminating unhealthy fats and eating healthy fats.
6. Eating organic and sustainable and when possible grass-fed animal proteins in moderation and occasionally. Eating organic, grass-fed dairy on occasion unless fermented.
7. Eating brain foods and spices.

Chapter 3: Looking for Mr. or Ms. Right

Jack and I both implemented the 7 Dementia Diet Principles and started to experience grand improvements in our health and therefore the quality of our lives. I then started to research into finding the right doctor or naturopath to design a vitamin and supplement regime for Jack to support our diet. When I mentioned to our doctor that we were considering the advice of a naturopath to formulate a vitamin regime for Jack, the doc declared, "Why would you do that? They are all quacks!"

One of Jack's friends highly recommended a naturopath in Michigan. Before booking an appointment, I looked this naturopath up on YouTube.com and watched a few of his videos. He certainly seemed legitimate and knowledgeable. But like our doctor, he voiced negativity toward traditional medicine, describing physicians as idiots and quacks.

We are cautious of anyone who negates others. When you point your finger at someone you have three fingers pointing back at yourself, Jack says. We also have always believed in living a healthy lifestyle, eating properly, exercising and also embracing traditional Western medicine when absolutely necessary. We refused to choose a single philosophy, to follow only this or that.

There had to be some expert in our province who believed in both an allopathic and naturopathic approach, I thought. I kept researching and prayed to the Great Creator. My prayer was answered.

I discovered Dr. Mordy Levy.

http://www.drlevy.ca

On his website I saw that not only did Dr. Levy support our own philosophy, he had 3 professional doctorate degrees! He was a medical doctor (MD), a chiropractor (DC) and a naturopathic doctor (ND). In fact, Dr. Levy is currently the only Canadian medical doctor (perhaps even internationally) that has obtained doctorates in three separate and unique health care professions (Chiropractic-1997, Medicine-2006, Naturopathic Medicine-2011) all from accredited, in residence universities.

His practice is north of Toronto, Ontario, Canada, about one and a half hour's drive from our home. And we didn't have to continue driving to Toronto each time because Dr. Levy conducted appointments via video conferencing. In fact, he sees patients from across the globe, thanks to today's advanced technology.

Jack had his first appointment with Dr. Levy. He never negates other physicians, ideals or philosophies. He is passionate and focuses on integrative and functional medicine.

We've never looked back. Dr. Levy ran extensive tests on Jack (blood, urine, and stool) looking for potential dysfunctions, which may have been contributing factors to the dementia (food reactions [IgG, IgE], nutritional deficiencies, toxic bioaccumulation, chronic latent infections, gut function, detoxification pathways, etc.)

Dr. Levy believes in a patient-centered approach and an Integrative and Functional Medicine Model (IFM) of health care. This means he implements evidence-based natural medical alternatives when indicated, in addition to enhancing function (hence functional medicine) by understanding physiopathology and treating mechanism(s) of disease processes, before they are pathological.

According to Dr. Levy, medicine should be holistic yet individualized and personalized. He says every patient is unique. This is opposite of the "disease-centered model of conventional medicine" implemented throughout North American in the health care systems. The patient-centered and whole health approach takes into consideration issues that may impact a person's overall whole health and wellness and therefore may have a direct or even indirect effect on their ability to cope with certain illnesses or disease processes.

*"You treat a disease, you win, you lose. You treat a person,
I guarantee you, you'll win, no matter what the outcome."*
--Dr. Patch Adams, MD

Dr. Levy says,
*"The human body is the most intriguing biological entity there is,
composed of many organ systems, subsystems, tissues, cells,
particles and sub-particles.
Furthermore, if you zoom into one area, you might miss the big
picture. This reductionist model of care is a serious shortcoming in
today's health care. Currently, we have many specialists and a
shrinking population of general practitioners. If someone has a
hormonal issue she is referred to an endocrinologist. If a patient
has a stomach concern, he is referred to a gastroenterologist, etc.
In my opinion we need more holistic generalists that assess the
entire patient as a whole, connects the dots between various
systems, and treats mechanism(s) of disease(s)."*

The combination of Jack taking the dementia medication and incorporating the 7 Dementia Diet Principles and the prescribed and individualized vitamin and supplement regime, designed by and under Dr. Levy's care that has added tremendous quality to Jack's current life and to his state of mind, body and spirit.

Jack says, "I feel normal again. I'm myself."

I have personally witnessed and viewed Jack's return to himself. Our lives are now filled with surprising, everyday mini-miracles.

Mind Returns:

Jack's clarity of mind has greatly improved, as well. He is now handling his daily finances, albeit slowly, and has even found some of his own mistakes. He now reads Vanity Fair and the newspaper regularly, albeit slowly. He is back to signing his own signature to documents. At the neurologist's office he initially improved in the clock-drawing test by two points. (The clock drawing test, used as a cognitive screening instrument, taps into

23

a wide range of cognitive abilities, such as executive functions. It is used for detecting early signs of dementia as well as progressing symptoms (as was the case with Jack). The test uses a simple scoring system with emphasis on the qualitative aspects of clock drawing.

The neurologist had Jack draw a clock by hand on a large piece of paper. He was then told to draw the face of a clock and put the numbers in the correct positions. He was then asked to draw the hands to indicate the time of ten minutes to eleven, for example. The neurologist then accessed and scored his efforts. To score, the neurologist assigned points for each part of the drawing:

- 1 point for a closed circle
- 1 point for properly placed numbers
- 1 point for including all twelve numbers
- 1 point for properly placed hands)

Two points may not seem like much, but they are two points heading in the right direction. These points are scientific proof that Jack is returning back to himself in some cognitive ways.

We like to watch Apple TV for Netflix and YouTube. The Apple TV remote is small and narrow with all operations performed from one button. It was too difficult for Jack to use. He would sit in front of the blank TV and patiently wait for me to come into the room to turn on the TV and use the remote to search for a movie for him. After a month on his vitamin/supplement regime, Jack was snatching the remote off the bedside table, and using the search engine to spell out movies, comedy shows and documentaries. A simple function that I use every day and take for granted. But in Jack's case, this was a mini miracle. An everyday mini-miracle.

Our first date took place at a Japanese restaurant. We both love sushi. Jack would handle chopsticks like they belonged to his hand. Before the Dementia Diet, Jack was unable to hold the chopsticks properly, often dropping pieces of his sushi rolls onto his plate. He was frustrated and annoyed. Dining out for sushi was no longer enjoyable for him. He reluctantly started to pick up each piece with his fingers. He also started to put the whole shrimp into his mouth, rather than biting down to cut off the hardened tail. This wasn't a good-day or bad-day change. It was a progressing decline of this simple skill of using chopsticks. A simple skill he used to immensely enjoy.

After being on the Dementia Diet, which also included his physician prescribed vitamin and supplement regime, Jack began to hold his chopsticks like fingers again. And using the chopsticks he could pick up small portions of rice and knew enough to bite off the shrimp tail. He is back to enjoying sushi again.

Body Strength and Health Returns:

Jack's strength and endurance have greatly improved. Before the Dementia Diet I would have to help him lift the garbage bag to the end of the driveway on garbage day. He now carries the bag himself. Before the Dementia Diet Jack would either work out at the gym with weights or instead swim laps in the pool. One or the other. This routine was also predicated on whether he was suffering from arthritic pain in his hip and knees that day. On one day his hip would hurt. On another day either knee would be arthritic and throbbing. He was often tired. After six weeks on the diet, Jack began working out at the gym more consistently with fewer days off for rest (rather than for pain). He now lifts weights and swims on the same days. He swims forty-four to fifty-three lengths on an average of two and sometimes three times per week. His workouts, in general, have increased to five to six times per week with almost no down time due to arthritic pain. He is an inspiration to our family and friends.

Posture and Motion Movement Returns:

My walking companion and friend Eleanor had not seen Jack on the walking trail for about four months. It was during this time that he had begun his vitamin regime. One day when he came walking with us, Eleanor noticed an unprecedented return in his walking ability. She said Jack was no longer hunched over and scuffling as he walked. Instead, his back was upright and he was taking normal strides. I noticed this too, once Eleanor brought it to my attention. In spending so much time with Jack I had not noticed this improvement myself. His walking normally and the use of the Apple TV remote were more than small improvements. They are restorations of body and coordination functions.

Spirit Returns:

Jack's spirit is healthy. I believe this is the case because we have created ourselves as partners in the Dementia Diet. The Dementia Diet is a way of living, an attitude and a commitment to something far greater than ourselves. It's for you if you are a caregiver, as much as it is for the one you love who lives with dementia. It's for you and your family.

I once heard the old adage, "There's your plan and there is God's plan and your plan doesn't matter." We accept the Great Creator's plan for our lives with Alzheimer's as our life experiment. It is a journey to embrace and enhance our own health and quality of lives, all the while being focused on making a difference for others. We hope this book makes a difference for you. If you are moved to change even one aspect of your diet and lifestyle to improve health and quality of life for yourself or for someone you love, then we will have succeeded. It is living in this way that keeps Jack (and myself) focused on the mission, on others, and on something greater than ourselves. It allows us to rise above seeing ourselves as hostages, as victims of this disease.

This is not to say that Jack's days are easy and stress free. And therefore my days are also not easy or stress free. Jack has Alzheimer's. As his caregiver, sometimes I get quiet moments alone that suddenly fill up with overwhelming fear. I then fantasize about running away. But then the moment passes and I move on. We both have good days and bad ones. Mostly, though, Jack's mood is steady with rare anger flare-ups. He is calm, peaceful and happy most of the time. He gets frustrated when he loses his wallet or cannot remember the names of his favourite actors or forgets his gym shorts at the health club or discovers that his missing wallet is in his jacket pocket, not the pocket of his pants. But the frustration quickly dissipates when he is reminded to accept 'forgetting' as part of his daily routine. I have become more patient. I regularly remind him that there's no upset, nowhere to get to, and that he needs to be kind to himself.

(As an aside, when Jack is agitated and angry it is usually a reflection of my own agitated or angry mood and how I have been impatient or frustrated in interacting and responding to him. I call this the "mirroring effect.")

For all these reasons, Jack does not suffer from depression often associated with dementia. He has a life mission that is so much larger than himself. We have a mission.

I also play CD's of Jack's favorite music in the car - Rock and Roll tunes from the 50's while we drive. He loves Fats Domino, the Platters, Roy Orbison, Little Richard, and Elvis Presley and others. It is absolutely amazing and transformational to see how music, such as masterful piano playing, or an angelic or velvety voice or sexy saxophone will move Jack to tears of joy. The songs send him back to his teenage memories of the places and people he loved.

He dances in the passenger seat, something completely of out character for my rough and tumble Navy SEAL. In getting out of the car he dances through the parking lot on his way into the pet shop for kitty litter. Jack is physically and spiritually moved by music.

Since his diagnoses, music has become an integral part of our lives. Incorporating music is part of creating this state of living in the moment, moment by moment, with peace of mind.

Don't Be Overwhelmed!

Don't be overwhelmed by all the changes in diet and health Jack has made in his life.

Incorporate the Dementia Diet at your own pace. Start slowly. We do not advocate the cold turkey approach.

We advocate that you get into action, start by finding a physician to put you on an individualized vitamin and supplement regime. Remember Dr. Levy sees patients across the globe. I highly recommend his services.

http://www.drlevy.ca

By implementing even just one or two of these principles, you will notice a grand return in your overall mind, body and spirit. My suggestion is that you begin with reducing and eventually eliminating refined sugar from your diet and moving to gluten-free whole foods.

Jack embraced the Dementia Diet like a Navy SEAL. I am so moved by who he is as a leader in his own life and in the lives of others. Jack is my inspiration. He is focused, consistent, disciplined and most importantly, highly coachable! He does exactly what Dr. Levy tell him. He follows the diet religiously. He is committed. After all, just as it was in Vietnam, his life is at stake.

Let's look at the Dementia Diet more closely...

Chapter 4: Sugar

I love sugar. As an author of cookbooks, I have always chosen classic ingredients for my dishes to produce the best results, texture and flavor. I use butter and I use sugar. But on the Dementia Diet sugar is not optimal.

The consumption of too much sugar not only makes us fat and wreaks havoc on our liver, but also triggers an immune response that results in inflammation and tissue damage in the body and inflammation in the brain, thus impairing mental function. Excess sugar has also been linked to diabetes and heart disease, both of which are linked to dementia. Sugar may also reduce the production of a protein called brain-derived neurotrophic factor (BDNF).

Since 1970 obesity rates have doubled and rates of diabetes have tripled. Not surprising. North Americans consume about 22 to 26 teaspoons of sugar per day in beverages and foods. That equates to about 130 pounds of sugar per year. And surprisingly it's quite easy to consume 22 to 26 teaspoons per day because sugar is buried (some might say strategically) in our favorite savory and sweet foods.

The Mayo Clinic published a study in the *Journal of Alzheimer's Disease* in 2012, showing that individuals who consume a high-carb diet have an increased risk for mild cognitive impairment, as high as 89%. This is in contrast to those who ate a high-fat diet, whose risk decreased by 44%. In 2011 Dr. Barnes and Yaffe (from the University of California, San Francisco) published a study in *Lancet Neurology* revealing that, in the United States, about 54% of Alzheimer's disease cases could have been prevented through lifestyle changes, such as exercise, weight loss, and in controlling hypertension.

The Bliss Point:

Food manufacturers are masters of the science of taste, texture and flavor and they surely know how to make their products taste good (some might say addictive).

The chorda tympani branch of the facial nerve carries our sensations of taste. We're born with a natural and instinctive ability to distinguish five basic tastes for survival - sourness, saltiness, bitterness, umami (roundness and depth of flavor) and sweetness.

Taste Sensations:

We crave these taste sensations, which in turn keep us alive. We love sour foods like lemons and limes, for example. They contain vitamins and minerals to ward off diseases like scurvy. By the same token, foods that sour (like milk) can make us sick which could lead to death. Our instinctive understanding of sourness keeps us alive.

We crave saltiness so our bodies do not dehydrate and cause death. Foods with bitterness like walnuts are loaded with vitamins and minerals that ward off diseases like cancer. Bitterness is also the taste sensation of most poisons. We have the instinctive ability to stay away from foods that taste bitter, which could lead to death. Bitterness is an instinctive survival mechanism.

Umami is the Japanese word for 'yummy' and refers to both simple and complex glutamate. Glutamate is found naturally in foods like potatoes. But it is also the source of increased flavor in foods that undergo slow cooking (ketchup), fermentation (cheese and soy sauce), ripening (cheese), or aging (beef).

Foods with complex glutamate are often fatty, like cheese and beef.

These five taste sensations, along with fattiness, are often combined to become the key ingredients in comfort foods. Mac and cheese is high in saltiness, umami and fattiness. Then we like to add a dollop of more umami and sweetness in the form of ketchup. Ice cream is also high in fattiness and sweetness and a popular comfort food.

We often eat comfort foods to ease our emotions and to ease stress. Nowadays our lives are fundamentally stressful. This is especially the case if you are a caregiver or a person with dementia.

In eating comfort food, we feel a sense of calm, of comfort. Why? Because instinctively the comfort food has told our brain that we are ultimately okay...we will survive.

Along with sourness, saltiness and bitterness, we're born with an instinctive love of sweetness. Mother's milk is sweet. When born we taste mother's milk for the first time and crave more. This keeps us alive, a survival mechanism.

Flavor Sensations:

We also have flavor sensations. We develop them after birth.

Flavor sensations include the taste sensations (sourness, sweetness, bitterness, saltiness and umami) plus two other groups: the trigeminal and retro-nasal sensations. These groups include the flavors of spiciness, fruitiness and fattiness.

The trigeminal nerve is responsible for the sensations of pain and burn, touch and temperature that can assault our mouth, and that we detect as warning signs of a variety of potentially harmful stimuli.

As well, the trigeminal nerve allows us to experience the positive effects of chemosensory irritations in beverages and foods. The spiciness or pleasant pain and burn of cayenne, the effervescence of champagne and the carbonation in soda aren't tastes, but chemosensory irritations - flavors - that many people enjoy and crave.

Retro-nasal olfaction is the perception of odors from inside the mouth. When we chew and swallow foods, the odors produced are forced behind the palate up into the nasal cavity.

The trigeminal input helps the brain determine whether an odor came into the nasal cavity via the nose (ortho-nasal) or mouth (retro-nasal).

Born neutral to odors, we learn to like or dislike them based on our experiences and their effect on us. We enjoy certain foods because of the odors experienced from inside our mouth, such as the fruitiness in fresh fruit. We also enjoy the odor and mouth feel of butter, olive oil and other fatty ingredients. On a negative note, if a food or beverage once made us sick to our stomach, it may smell disgusting to us for the rest of our life.

Back to Sugar: The Bliss Point

Let's get back to one survival taste sensation – sugar. Food and beverage manufacturers employ sensory scientists and chemists. They understand our survival mechanisms. That's why sugar is essential in approximately 99 percent of all processed foods, both sweet and savory kinds. It adds flavor. It caters to our survival need. It drives the taste in most processed products and its high level found in each product is no accident.

Many food companies search for what is referred to as the 'bliss point' in products. The bliss point is the amount of an ingredient like sugar, salt, or fat within a processed food to optimize its palatability. It's the point where the majority of people like the product the most. Once a product's bliss point is discovered, the product is ready for large-scale manufacturing.

In creating and implementing a diet to slow the progression of Jack's dementia, to reverse symptoms and to return him back to himself, thus enhancing the quality of his life, my greatest breakthroughs and therefore changes were in taking the time to read food labels. I have been religiously reducing the amount of hidden sugar we were both consuming daily. As a side benefit to increasing brain health, we have both lost undesirable weight.

I was shocked by how much hidden sugar we consumed without knowing it. Sugar is a part of almost all processed foods. It's in ketchup, peanut butter, mayonnaise, salad dressing, barbecue sauce, relish, cereal, and spaghetti sauce, to name but a few. My favorite fat-free plain Greek yogurt...plain yogurt... has sugar.

Four grams equals one teaspoon of sugar. Did you know that a 'healthy' protein bar eaten to replace breakfast can contain up to five different types of sugars? Read the label. Here you may find a single ingredient list made up of sugar, evaporated cane juice, invert sugar, corn syrup, and barley malt syrup.

Let's look at a condiment that we keep handy in the refrigerator - - ketchup. One tablespoon (three teaspoons) of ketchup possesses one teaspoon of sugar. One third of ketchup's make up is sugar! With every order of French fries Jack and I used to consume about two tablespoons of ketchup and therefore two teaspoons of sugar. French fries with sugar!

My favorite company offers 'no sugar added' with only one gram of sugar in one tablespoon of ketchup. So where's the bliss point? It's in the sodium content, of course. While low in sugar, this product has 200 grams of sodium in every tablespoon of ketchup. If you purchase the low sodium version, wanting to prevent or manage high blood pressure, you ingest five grams of sugar in every tablespoon of ketchup. Sugar is a main culprit for high blood pressure, as well. The only ketchup low in sugar and sodium is the homemade kind. We have a tasty homemade ketchup recipe in our book called Dementia Diet: Everyday Mini-Miracles Cookbook available through Amazon.

So, the point to remember is that every processed food has its bliss point in salt, sugar or fat, whether it's labeled as healthy or not.

Dr. Robert H. Lustig, MD, is an American pediatric endocrinologist and Professor of Clinical Pediatrics from the University of California in San Francisco. He is renowned as the 'man who believes sugar is poison.' According to Dr. Lustig, there are 30% more obese people on the planet then there are undernourished ones. He stated in 2011, that there were 366 million diabetics on the earth (according to statistics gathered by the International Diabetes Federation). Dr. Lustig also claims that diabetes costs the United States $244 billion dollars per year.

Over the last fifty years, as obesity has dramatically inclined, so too has type 2 diabetes. Numerous studies have proven that individuals with diabetes, especially type 2, are at risk of heart disease and stroke and have a lower level of cognitive function and are at a higher risk for developing dementia.

As stated earlier, one of the hallmarks of Alzheimer's is brain starvation also referred to as type 3 diabetes. Type 3 diabetes is an extension of type 1 and type 2. Type 3 follows a similar pathophysiology as type 2, but in the brain. Insulin is needed to help the neurons in the brain absorb glucose for healthy functioning. Insulin-resistant brain cells can lead to Alzheimer's.

People with insulin resistance, those with type 2 diabetes, also have an increased risk of developing Alzheimer's, estimated to be between 50% and 65% higher.

Jack's Return to Well-Being:

The reduction and we strive for the elimination of sugar from our diet has had the greatest impact on Jack's health and mood. Drastically reducing sugar intake has added to the clarity (or less fogginess) of Jack's mind. He also experiences far less arthritic flare-ups. And he is now keenly aware of how within hours of eating sugar, his hip and knee becomes inflamed and aches with arthritic pain. Once addicted to ice cream, Jack is now more interested in being pain free.

I remember an incident that occurred about ten years ago. I was working in the kitchen when Jack came in. His face was red and the veins were popping out of his neck. He was enraged. I was concerned and said, "What's wrong?"

With shaking shoulders he yelled, "Someone didn't do the laundry." (That someone was me, of course.)

Jack is an edgy character. His favorite line is, "I have no commitment to being a nice guy."

(As an aside, Jack is committed to being authentic, to being himself. He also happens to have a deep love for his children, cats and human beings of all cultures, races, religions, shapes and sizes.)

This outburst was far more dramatic than usual. I replied, "Okay, so what? You act as though you just learned I skinned your cat alive."

He left the room ranting about the laundry.

A few hours later I was rummaging through the freezer and noticed that an entire tub of chocolate ice cream was missing. I asked Jack about it and he admitted to having consumed the entire tub that afternoon.

I started to link that there may be a direct relationship between Jack's sugar intake, a dramatic increase in his blood sugar level, and his angry outbursts.

Now, on the Dementia Diet, Jack no longer eats store-bought ice cream. I make a homemade version with unsweetened almond milk, stevia, bitter chocolate and toasted pecans. It's a real treat for him. We eat homemade frozen fruit pops regularly. I blend together coconut milk and lime juice. Or I make homemade frozen yogurt using So Delicious (dairy free coconut yogurt), frozen mixed berries and Stevia for sweetness. We have found a local vendor who makes on-the-spot frozen yogurt with no added sugar and fresh fruit.

Since minimizing his consumption of sugar, Jack is pain free, calm and peaceful most of the time.

Understanding Sugar: Glucose and Fructose:

Medical research has linked sugar to disease for decades. Sugar has empty calories and is believed to be poisonous to our health.

Every granule of sugar can be broken down into two primary molecules. They are glucose and fructose.

Glucose is found in fruits, such as blueberries, raisins and honey and from starches like potatoes. It is sometimes referred to as 'blood sugar.' Because glucose is absorbed directly by the body, it rapidly increases our blood sugar levels, giving it a high glycemic index.

Fructose is found in natural compounds like fruits and vegetables, but also in processed foods.

Glucose and fructose are metabolized differently in the body. When they separate in our stomach, glucose becomes fuel, immediately feeding our muscles, brain, and the whole body.

The New England Journal of Medicine published an article entitled *Glucose Levels and Risk of Dementia*. In the article it states that, "the results of studies assessing the association between obesity or diabetes and the risk of dementia have been mixed. It is imperative to understand the potential consequences of the obesity and diabetes epidemics for the incidence of dementia. Any effects that obesity has on the risk of dementia are likely to include effects on metabolism. We evaluated extensive longitudinal clinical data from a prospective cohort with research-quality case ascertainment to test the hypothesis that glucose levels are associated with the risk of dementia."

The abstract's conclusions state, "our results suggest that higher glucose levels may be a risk factor for dementia, even among persons without diabetes." (Funded by the National Institute of Health.)

Fructose, on the other hand, can only be metabolized in the liver. And it is in the liver that problems arise. When the liver is forced to metabolize excess fructose, it turns into liver fat. This is a precursor to non-alcoholic fatty liver disease. Having a fatty liver increases the risk of metabolic diseases, such as abdominal obesity, high cholesterol and triglycerides, high blood pressure, insulin resistance, blood clots and inflammation. Excess fructose is also believed to increase uric acid (which causes gout), cancer and type 2 diabetes. Too much fructose in the liver also shuts down the part of the brain that tells us that our stomach is full. This leads to excess eating and obesity. A vicious cycle.

Keep in mind that this does not mean that the fructose in natural fruits and vegetables is bad for us. Fruits and vegetables are made up of water, fructose, fiber, minerals and vitamins. We would have to eat a ridiculous amount of fruit or vegetables to reach a harmful fructose level in our liver. It is the fructose of 'added sugar' to processed foods to create the bliss point that contributes to fatty liver disease.

Sugar Reduces BDNF: Brain-Derived Nerve Growth Factor:

As stated, sugar may reduce the production of a protein called brain-derived neurotrophic factor (BDNF). It is also referred to as the 'miracle-grow' for the brain.

Research shows that a high-sugar diet reduces the production of a brain chemical called BDNF. Without this protein, our brain fails to form new memories and cannot learn anything new. Or said another way, the abundant presence of BDNF in the body and brain predicts ease of learning and memory retention.

Studies have also shown that levels of BDNF are low in people with diabetes or pre-diabetes. Research has also linked low BDNF to dementia and depression. Some experts believe that BDNF may be a key factor when it comes to preventing, slowing and perhaps playing a part in one-day curing dementia and Alzheimer's disease.

Incorporate Omega 3s In Your Diet:

Foods high in Omega 3 fats (with a lower Omega 6 fatty acid ratio), regular physical exercise, and quality sleep all improve our production of BDNF. We can also obtain more BDNF through Omega 3 in vitamin form. I advocate that you speak to your specialist or doctor before implementing vitamins into your diet if you suffer from any form of degenerative disease or are on medication(s). Medications and vitamins and natural herbs can have negative interactions.

As stated by famous neurologist, Dr. David Perlmutter, author of the bestselling book *Grain Brain*, "One of the key factors that correlates levels of DHA to brain health and disease resistance is DHA's ability to turn on the brain's growth hormone called BDNF."

Omega 3 fats are part of the polyunsaturated fat family. They are sometimes referred to as poly fats.

The most nutrient dense forms of Omega 3s are found in flax seeds and walnuts. Very good sources are sardines, salmon, and beef, Brussels sprouts, cauliflower and mustard seeds. Good sources include shrimp, winter squash, broccoli, cod, collard greens, spinach, summer squash, raspberries, kale, green beans, and strawberries, to name a few.

If you are vegan, you can obtain your Omega 3's through sea plants, leafy greens (spinach, broccoli, kale), legumes (kidney, navy, pinto, lima), nuts, seeds and citrus fruits, melons and cherries and ground flaxseed. General vegetarians can get their Omega 3 fats from these same foods listed above as well as from dairy products (eggs, milk and cheese and yogurt). The key is to ensure that these food items derive from animals that have grazed on grass rather than on grain and corn. The old adage, "You are what you eat," also applies to cows, goats and sheep.

For the rest of us non-vegetarians we can also obtain our Omega 3s from all the foods listed above, as well as from grass fed meats.

So, when it comes to preparing Jack's diet, I use natural low glycemic sweeteners like stevia (covered in the next chapter) and also ensure our diet is packed with foods high in Omega 3s. I add MCT oil (Medium Chain Triglyceride oil) , a liquid form, to sauces, soups, vinaigrettes, to his organic peanut butter and anywhere else where oil is required. It's loaded in Omega 3! I add the oil "after" the cooking process is completed so it retains all of its nutrients. We also take an Omega 3 supplement. (This is covered in Chapter 9.)

Diabetes and Dementia:

Diabetes is a metabolic disorder. It means the body cannot properly store and use sugar (glucose) for energy. The sugar comes from food, but is also made by the liver. Your blood carries the sugar to every cell in your body, including your brain. To use sugar (glucose) the body requires a hormone called insulin. Insulin regulates blood sugar by stimulating the removal of sugar from the blood and taking it up to the muscles, liver, fat cells, body, and brain.

When you eat carbohydrates like pasta and white bread, they are turned into sugar almost as fast as if you were to drink a bottle of sweetened iced tea. This is because normal starch, made up of tangled chains of glucose sugar molecules, is quickly and easily broken down into single sugar molecules and absorbed by the blood stream. If you don't burn off this sugar, it is stored as fat.

Bread and pasta are examples of digestible starches. Digestible starches cause a rise in blood sugar, which causes a spike in insulin levels. As blood sugar levels rise, the pancreas produces insulin, a hormone that prompts cells throughout the body to absorb blood sugar for energy. As cells absorb blood sugar, levels of sugar in the bloodstream fall. To correct this fall of the blood sugar level, the pancreas then makes a hormone called glucagon which signals the liver to release more stored sugar to compensate. The toxic interaction of insulin and glucagon begins, ensuring that cells throughout the body, especially in the brain, have a steady supply of blood sugar.

Over time, however, this fluctuation and wear and tear on the body becomes too much. The body cannot make enough or use enough insulin. It's called insulin resistance. Insulin resistance, also called metabolic syndrome, puts you on the path toward pre-diabetes or type 2 diabetes.

In an article published on the Alzheimer's Association website and according to the American Diabetes Association, 27% of people aged sixty-five and older in the United States have diabetes and about half have pre-diabetes. Numerous studies have found that individuals with diabetes, especially type 2, have a lower level of cognitive function and are at higher risk for dementia than individuals without diabetes. As mentioned earlier, as high as 65%. This is not a surprising percentage when you consider that the average person consumes about 135 to 180 pounds of sugar per year.

The article goes on to say that, *"In the October 2013 issue of the Journal of Alzheimer's Disease, researchers reported a strong correlation between Alzheimer's disease and high blood sugar levels. The study found that people with high blood sugar levels, such as those linked with type 2 diabetes, had a dramatic increase in a protein toxic to cells in the brain...A study published in the July 2013 issue of Alzheimer's & Dementia: The Journal of the Alzheimer's Association was the first to show that people in the early stages of type 2 diabetes have signs of brain dysfunction. Study participants showed high levels of insulin resistance in the brain and a reduced ability to use glucose to fuel normal brain function..."*

The list of published research studies and papers linking high blood sugar levels and type 2 diabetes to Alzheimer's and to other types of dementia is lengthy and growing.

If you are pre-diabetic or have diabetes, be sure to consult your physician before undertaking any new dietary plan.

In an organic nut shell:

a) All sugar is digested the same way.
b) Sugar causes inflammation in the body and brain.
c) Don't be fooled by food labels boasting healthy claims. Every processed food has a bliss point. Sugar is primarily the bliss point ingredient.
d) Refrain from eating refined sugar whenever possible.
e) Eating too much refined sugar may lead to diabetes, heart disease and dementia.
f) Keep your blood sugar level under control to protect your arteries and nerves and to prevent diabetes, heart disease, the loss of memory, and thinking skills.
g) Stop eating sugar (and definitely refined sugar) whenever possible to help prevent and reverse symptoms of dementia.
h) Increase your consumption of foods high in Omega 3 to increase your miracle-grow protein called BDNF, which is good for your brain.

Chapter 5: The Glycemic Index and Sugar Substitutes

What is the glycemic index?

The Glycemic Index (GI) is related to carbohydrates. Carbohydrates are found in fruits, vegetables, breads, cereals and grains, milk products, and foods containing sugars. Our body uses these carbohydrates (carbs) to make glucose, which acts as fuel. Our body either uses it immediately or stores it in our liver and muscles for when it will be required later on.

When carbohydrates are consumed, the GI measures how quickly sugar enters the bloodstream. If it enters too quickly, our brain signals our body to secrete a great amount of insulin. Insulin helps draw sugar out of the bloodstream by converting the excess into fat that is stored in the body. The greater the increase in blood sugar leads to a greater insulin release, which leads to more fat stored in the body. This leads to a sudden drop in the blood sugar level, which causes fatigue.

When confronted with whether or not to indulge in that chocolate bar or ice cream cone, we often rationalize that it's 'just one.' Or we say to ourselves, "I'll cut out sugar for the rest of the week." And then we don't. The challenge is that we don't experience the cause and effect of consuming foods with a high glycemic sugar index right away. Its effects creep up later in life in the form of diabetes, dementia, heart disease and other degenerative diseases.

Every carbohydrate has a Glycemic Index. Some are low while others may be moderate or high.

The GI is a number associated with a specific food, ranging from 0 to 100, and indicates the food's effect on our blood sugar level.

Here is a general breakdown:

Low (zero to 55)
Moderate (56 to 70)

High (Over 71)

The GI number helps us understand how our body breaks down carbohydrates... that is, carbohydrates minus the fiber content of a food. Fiber, protein and fat all slow down the entry of glucose from a food into the bloodstream.

The Glycemic Load:

Some foods cause quick and dramatic peaks (high glycemic foods) in blood glucose, while others do not (low to moderate glycemic foods). The lower the GI, the slower the effect of glucose on our blood sugar levels. One hundred equals pure glucose or sugar.

This is called the Glycemic Load (GL) and is probably more important than the GI as it takes into consideration how quickly a certain food converts to sugar (GI), as well as how much sugar a particular food contains. If a food is low in sugar it will have a low glycemic load.

Watermelon, for example, has a high glycemic index, but a low glycemic load for the amount consumed. Fructose, by contrast, has a low glycemic index, but can have a high glycemic load if a large quantity is consumed.

The glycemic index does not measure insulin production due to rises in blood sugar. Therefore two foods could have the same glycemic index, but produce different amounts of insulin. Or two foods could have the same glycemic load, but cause different insulin responses.

Foods containing wheat and gluten have a higher glycemic index than those that are gluten and wheat free. Inside the world of gluten-free, some flours, for example, have a lower glycemic index than others as well. So there is more to the science of going 'gluten-free' than just giving up wheat.

Legume, chickpea or soybean flour have a lower GI number than potato and corn flours.

Quinoa, basmati rice and sweet corn have moderate GI values. So consuming pasta and bread made from rice flour or buckwheat or quinoa can help satisfy your carbohydrate craving without spiking your blood sugar.

Sweeteners:

Chemically all sugars are much the same, whether they are refined or natural. Corn syrup, agave syrup, white or brown sugar, honey, molasses, and maple syrup -- they are all high in fructose and are processed by the liver in the same way.

That's why it is important to consume sugar in small amounts or perhaps only on special occasions. While at home, Jack and I refrain from refined and hidden sugars as much as possible. But if we are dining out or at other people's homes or celebrating a special occasion we will share dessert. Again, the Dementia Diet is not about sacrifice. It's about discipline and consistency on a regular basis.

How about artificial sweeteners? In my opinion, it's best to refrain from artificial sweeteners altogether. Recent studies show a link between artificial sweeteners and weight gain. It appears that if we know a specific food is low in sugar and calories, we tend to eat more of it, thus gaining an increase of calories from its other ingredients. Weight gain can lead to obesity. Obesity can lead to type 2 diabetes. Type 2 diabetes can lead to dementia.

There are a few sweeteners found in nature that are actually good for our health. They are low on the glycemic index, low in calories, and low in fructose. They also taste extremely sweet and delicious. And, unlike sugar, they have some form of trace vitamins and minerals. These sweeteners are pleasurable alternatives.

They are: Stevia, Erythritol, Xylitol, and Yacon Syrup.

I've also included other natural sweeteners and their glycemic index if you find that you simply cannot give up sugar to substitute it for one of the top four.

Stevia: Glycemic Index 0
1 tablespoon of sugar = ¼ teaspoon of stevia powdered extract = 6 to 7 drops of Stevia concentrated liquid

Personally we are loyal stevia customers. I add it to tea and coffee, homemade frozen yogurts, and desserts. It took a while but our palates are now conditioned for stevia instead of sugar.

Stevia is a "sweet" sugar substitute. In fact, it is 200 times sweeter than sugar! It has been a sweet staple in the South American diet for centuries. With zero calories and a glycemic index of zero, stevia has become a popular substitute for diabetics and those on a low glycemic diet. While it derives from a plant, stevia is highly refined so might also fit into the 'artificial' sweetener category. In my opinion its benefits far out weight its disadvantages when it comes to preventing and slowing the progression of dementia. Cheap versions of stevia can possess a bitter after taste. So be sure to purchase one that is reasonably priced and tastes great. Stevia is not a good substitute for sugar in baking. It comes in various forms, such as granulated and fluffy or concentrated, for example.

Raw Yacon: Glycemic Index 1
3/4 cup = 1 cup of sugar

Extracted from the Yacon plant (a tuber), this South American sweetener has half the calories of sugar and a high concentration of indigestible inulin fiber, which means it breaks down slowly in the body. It is also high in potassium, calcium, phosphorous, iron and twenty amino acids! And, just as important, Yacon is low in fructose. It also contains fructooligosaccharides (pronounced fruc-tol-ago-sac-a-rides), which functions as soluble fiber that feeds the good bacteria in the intestines. Research has shown that this natural sweetener has caused significant weight loss in overweight women.

Sugar Alcohols Ending in 'itrol':
Erythritol: Glycemic Index 0
1 tbsp. = 1 tbsp. of sugar

Erythritol (pronounced ur-wreath-ra-tall) is a sugar alcohol found naturally in fruits. This sweetener also has a low glycemic index, has four calories per gram and has no effect on biomarkers like cholesterol or triglycerides. It does have a slightly bitter after taste.

Somewhat less sweet than sugar, Erythritol adds stability and shelf life to baked goods and barely alters the texture of the goods. Its brand names include ZSweet, Sweet Simplicity, and Zero.

*Xylitol: Glycemic Index 7
1 cup = 1 cup of sugar

I've tried Xylitol (pronounced Zi-la-tall) several times. It is readily available in bulk food stores and on Amazon. It looks and acts like sugar. The only issue I have is that it is not as sweet as stevia. So it's psychologically deceiving to put two teaspoons of Xylitol into my large almond milk latte and have it taste only half as sweet as expected. Unlike Stevia, Xylitol has less bitter taste.

Xylitol is a naturally occurring sugar alcohol found in fruits and vegetables. But it is neither sugar nor alcohol. Once extracted and processed, Xylitol becomes a white, crystalline granule sweetener that can replace sugar. It is low on the glycemic index and so does not cause a spike in the blood sugar and actually helps to reduce sugar cravings. It stabilizes both insulin and hormone levels. Xylitol reduces the risk of cavities, improves bone density and increases the absorption of B-vitamins and calcium. The majority of Xylitol comes from China and derives from corn. However, Canada (my country) boasts about producing the finest Xylitol extracted entirely from North American hardwood trees.

Its brand names include XyloSweet, XyloPure, Miracle Sweet, and Nature's Provision.

Agave Nectar: Glycemic Index 15
1 ¼ cups = 1 cup of sugar

I love the taste of Agave, especially for baking. I just find it too expensive and simply not sweet enough for our liking. The Aztecs loved agave syrup, considering it a gift from the Gods that derives from the Blue Agave cactus plant. This is the same syrup that is fermented to produce tequila. Similar to honey in flavor, agave is half as sweet as sugar. This Aztec sweetener is rich in vitamins E, C, and D, calcium, iron, zinc and magnesium. When baking use ¾ cup of agave syrup to every one cup of white sugar.

Lucuma: Glycemic Index 25
1 cup = 2 cups sugar

This substitute is made from the Peruvian lucuma fruit. Its dried version is milled into a fine powder. Thus it retains all of its natural beta carotene and B-vitamins. Lucuma tastes much like maple. One tablespoon of sugar has about forty-eight calories. Lucuma has sixty! BUT...you tend to use half as much because of its intense sweet taste! It's a great substitute in recipes calling for brown sugar. Lucuma is also high in iron, zinc, potassium, calcium, magnesium, vitamin B3, beta carotene, and fiber.

Brown Rice Sugar: Glycemic Index 25
1 1/3 cups = 1 cup of sugar

This sweetener's name says it all. It is made from boiled rice and has a thick, gooey consistency. Some of its many health benefits include B5, vitamin K, niacin, and thiamin.

Coconut Palm Sugar: Glycemic Index 35
1 cup = 1 cup of brown sugar

Coconut palm sugar comes from the sap of the coconut tree. It has the same amount of calories as refined sugar but a lower glycemic index. This sweetener is also rich in magnesium, potassium, zinc and B vitamins.

Maple Syrup – Glycemic Index 54
¾ cup = 1 cup of sugar

Friends of mine, Jill and Robert Staples, have been producing maple syrup in my region, the Kawarthas and Northumberland County, for many years. In 1813 the original Staples wrote back to Ireland about the sweet sap from the maple trees and generations later every spring the whole Staples family become involved in the process of making maple syrup! They produce International award-winning maple syrup in different grades and tastes. Jill first told me that new studies suggest that Canadian maple syrup does not spike sugar levels and therefore is good for diabetics.

A recent study backs up Jill and Robert Staples' information. Researchers from the U.S., Canada, Mexico and Japan joined together on March 16, 2014 at the annual meeting of the American Chemical Society (ACS), in Dallas, Texas. They attended a full-day symposium devoted to a number of studies examining potential new health benefits found in maple syrup and other natural sweeteners. One study found that Canadian maple syrup does not cause the same spike in blood insulin levels as some other sugars in tests performed with laboratory animals. This new data shows promise for those with type 2 diabetes and metabolic syndrome, both of which can contribute to dementia.

Like growing and vinifying wine grapes, the business of tapping sugar maple trees for sap to be evaporated into syrup is truly a labor of love. It is a painstaking, hand-made process that takes about thirty to forty litres of sap to yield one litre of syrup.

In our province we currently have about fifty maple orchards. A maple orchard is a managed plantation of sugar maple and black maple trees grown to produce maple syrup.

Just as in the growing of wine grapes, the weather plays an important role in the production of maple sap. The best conditions are warm, sunny days followed by freezing nights. Poor weather conditions affect both the quality and quantity of sap.

Maple sap is about 97% water. Through boiling or reverse osmosis, the water is evaporated, transforming the sap into syrup.

The evaporation process develops the flavor and colour of the syrup. The colour of the syrup can be used as an indicator of flavor. In Canada we have various grades and several colour classes of maple syrup. The first grade is Canada No. 1, which includes extra light, light and medium. This syrup is light tasting and is often used on pancakes and waffles. Canadian No. 2 Amber, also called Ontario Amber, is darker and stronger tasting. Due to its intensity of flavor, this syrup is often used as a cooking ingredient.

If you must consume sugar, turn to maple syrup.

Raw Honey: Glycemic Index 62
¾ cup = 1 cup of sugar

If you must have some form of sugar, consider honey, as well. It possesses about twenty-two calories per teaspoon. As a result, people 'generally' consume about half as much. So it becomes a better caloric trade off. This sweetener is also less processed. The refining process strips out the vitamins, minerals, proteins, and fiber once found in the sugar cane. Hence sugar becomes empty calories.

Honey is anti-bacterial, anti-fungal and anti-viral. So the next time you have the flu or a bad cold, sip lemon-ginger tea with fresh lemon juice and fresh ginger, and use raw honey. Honey is also alkalizing for the body and aids in acid-indigestion. Research also shows raw honey reduces muscle cramps and cures insomnia. Vitamins B1, B2, B3, B5, B6, as well as vitamin C are found in honey, along with magnesium, potassium, calcium, sodium chlorine, copper, iron, manganese, zinc and phosphate. It's super healthy!

The biggest secret about raw honey? It helps to dissolve fat. In the morning consume one to two teaspoons of raw honey in warm water with fresh lemon.

Date Sugar: Glycemic Index 68
2/3 cup = 1 cup brown sugar

Made from dehydrated ground dates, this sugar is packed with nutritional benefits, such as potassium, calcium, iron, magnesium, phosphorus, zinc, iron, copper, manganese and selenium.

In an organic nut shell:

a) Sugar ultimately leads to brain starvation and inflammation.
b) All sugar, natural or artificial, is processed by the liver in the same way. Therefore refrain from cooking with and eating sugar as much as possible.
c) Avoid artificial sweeteners.
d) Choose low glycemic natural sweeteners like Stevia, Erythritol, Xylitol and Yacon Syrup.
e) Eat moderately foods with a high glycemic index.
f) When consuming healthy foods with a high glycemic index incorporate fat, fiber and/or protein to slow down the digestion of the sugar, thus keeping your blood sugar level from spiking.
g) If you eat bread, then choose low glycemic gluten-free breads made from rice, buckwheat or quinoa.

Chapter 6: Why Does the Dementia Diet Include Gluten-Free?

Simply said gluten causes inflammation of the body and the brain.

What is Gluten?

Gluten is a protein found in wheat, barley, and rye. It is a composite created when two proteins (glutenin and gliadin (pronounced glee-a-din)) are mixed with water and form hydrogen bonds, allowing them to form a sturdy network. Gluten creates structure. It allows bread to hold its shape, absorb moisture and become more elastic. It gives pasta that wonderful al dente texture. Flour has gluten. Flour is a hidden binding ingredient in many products such as soups, sauces, spices, gravies, and thickeners, and even in beer and liquor. Hence these products contain gluten.

Oats are gluten-free, but can be gluten contaminated. Most commercial oats are processed in facilities that also process wheat, barley, and rye. So if you have Celiac disease or are highly sensitive to gluten, refrain from eating oats, unless you know they are free of gluten contamination.

There are distinctions to be made between Celiac disease, wheat allergies and gluten intolerance and sensitivity.

Even if you do not suffer from Celiac disease or gluten intolerance or sensitivity, the elimination of wheat, rye and barley can be beneficial to your health and brain.

Super Glutens and Frankenwheat:

The wheat we consume today is not the same wheat consumed by our ancestors. Today's wheat is considered as a type of Frankenstein version of the original grain.

There are three cultivated wheat species. They are Diplois (pronounced dip-loyz), Diploid and Tetrapoid (pronounced tit-tra-poyd). Wheat varieties within each species have varying levels of the gluten proteins called gliadin and glutenin. Gliadin is the soluble element in gluten; glutenin is the insoluble one.

Those suffering from Celiac disease or gluten-intolerance are reacting to gliadin protein. Gliadin causes an inflammatory reaction as it comes into contact with the wall of the small intestine. This low-grade inflammation may go undetected for years before symptoms become obvious. This can cause a slow destruction of the healthy living tissues within the small intestine. Over time gliadin intolerance creates significant stress on the immune system.

About 2.6 million years ago our ancestors consumed a wild species of wheat called Einkorn. Einkorn (of the Diplois species) is non-genetically altered with fourteen chromosomes of gliadin.

In the 1950's scientists began crossbreeding and hybridizing wheat to make it hardier, shorter, and able to resist pests and diseases. As crop rotation was applied to long cultivated land, along with the use of fertilizers, yields of wheat increased. Wheat was required to feed larger populations across the globe. What we now know is that this morphing of wheat from its ancient form to its present version also introduced compounds believed to be unfriendly to the human digestive system.

Today's wheat variety (called bread or common wheat) and part of the Diploid species, is the most widely grown and used for the production of almost all commercial wheat products. Common wheat has strong and elastic gluten that enables its dough to trap carbon dioxide during leavening and is therefore beneficial in the making of baked products like bread. The issue is that common wheat has a grand total of forty-two chromosomes of gliadin -- not fourteen like its ancestral version.

Durum wheat (part of the Tetrapoid species) is used for making pasta and contains twenty-eight chromosomes of gliadin.

Durum and Bread wheat contain more than double and triple the amount of the protein gliadin as found in the ancient grain Einkorn. These hybridized and crossbred varieties are often referred to as 'super glutens' or 'Frankenwheats.'

Why should we care about the level of the protein gliadin in our breads and pastas? The reason is that high levels of gliadin are believed to trigger inflammation in the body. Inflammation then triggers insulin resistance, causing an increase in the appetite, gradual weight gain, and ultimately type 2 diabetes. We know that type 2 diabetes can cause dementia.

Research shows that super gluten wheat raises blood sugar levels, causing immunoreactive problems, inhibits the absorption of important minerals, and aggravates our intestines. These wheat are now believed by many scientists and experts to contribute to obesity, diabetes, heart disease, cancer, dementia, depression and a plethora of other illnesses.

(Keep in mind that there are researchers, scientists, physicians and experts on the other side of the argument who will adamantly argue that wheat does not lead to these health conditions. They believe that if you are not suffering from Celiac disease or gluten sensitivity, then removing it from the diet is unnecessary and even ludicrous.)

No source of Frankenwheat — not newly sprouted or in baked bread, pasta or pastries -- is good for us.

Other Grains with Gliadin Structures:

Rye and barley share similar gliadin structures to wheat. There is much controversy over corn. In relation to Celiac disease, corn has not been studied to the same extent as wheat. But thus far, studies show that corn proteins on the celiac intestine are safe.

Brain Inflammation:

"That gluten sensitivity is regarded as principally a disease of the small bowel is a historical misconception. Gluten sensitivity can be primarily and at times exclusively a neurological disease."

- Dr. Marios Hadjivassilou (Journal of Neurology, Neurosurgery & Psychiatry)

Dr. Rodney Ford, a New Zealand paediatrician and author of "The Gluten Syndrome," believes that gluten can make you sick in the head – literally. A gluten diet affects the brain and neurological tissues directly, he believes.

"Do you know that a teaspoon of gluten, if you have the gluten gene or gluten sensitivity, can cause brain inflammation that lasts up to 30 days? Do you know that if you have the gluten gene or gluten sensitivity, that if you eat gluten, it can decrease the blood supply to certain parts of the brain, by 35% to 40%?"

--Dr. Brian Roadhouse

According to Dr. Jay Sordean, Lac, OMD, QME, NRCT certified practitioner and author of "Superbrain," gluten sensitivity and food allergies can lead to leaky brain syndrome. Alzheimer's, dementia, brain damage, all decrease quality of life and abilities to function.

Dr. Sordean says, *"In talking about the health of the nervous system, the brain and the spinal cord, a diagnosis of a variety of different conditions requires a multi-step and comprehensive approach to figure out exactly what may be going on causing degeneration and a breakdown in the brain and nervous system. What might be damaging? The nerves? We are causing an overall metabolic breakdown. Not getting enough oxygen. Not getting enough energy to the nerves. Food allergies, as well as gluten sensitivity...*

Some people estimate that up to ¾ of the population has a gluten-sensitivity. This sensitivity can set up immunological reactions, in the small intestine, which breaks down that barrier which causes immunological reactions that reach all the way to the brain."

Celiac Disease and Diagnosis:

Celiac disease is a lifelong autoimmune response caused by intolerance to gluten. It is life threatening. It is believed that one in every 100 people have this condition. There are no typical signs and symptoms of Celiac disease. However, symptoms include bloating, diarrhea, nausea, gas, constipation, tiredness, headaches, muscle cramps, sudden weight loss, hair loss, anemia, osteoporosis, and abdominal pain.

Sometimes people with Celiac disease have no abdominal symptoms at all. Instead, a person can suffer irritability, joint pain, muscle cramps, mouth sores, tingling in the feet, or a rash called dermatitis herpetiformis – an itchy, blistering skin disease. It is estimated that about ten percent of patients with Celiac disease also have this skin disorder.

A blood test showing an elevated level of antibodies is an indication of Celiac disease. This indicates that one's immune system recognizes gluten as a foreign substance and increases the number of antibodies to fight it.

After the blood tests, the doctor will perform intestinal tissue testing to check for damage to the villi. A thin, flexible tube is inserted through the mouth, esophagus and stomach and into the small intestine. The doctor then takes a small tissue sample. The tiny, hair-like projections from the small intestine that absorb vitamins, minerals and other nutrients will provide the necessary information.

After undergoing medical examination, a gluten-free trial period can confirm the diagnosis. It's important that the medical examination is done first. Otherwise, the diet may have an impact on the results of the blood test and biopsies. They may appear normal and without any complications even if the patient is positive with Celiac disease.

Wheat Allergy:

Wheat allergies are also an immune response to wheat and to gluten. It is one of the most common allergies in children. It is often confused with Celiac disease or gluten sensitivity. A wheat allergy shows different symptoms. Symptoms include swelling, itching or irritations of the mouth or throat, hives, rashes of the skin, nasal congestion, itchy and watery eyes, difficulty breathing, cramps, nausea or vomiting, diarrhea and anaphylaxis (tightening of the throat, fast heartbeat, difficulty breathing, trouble swallowing, dizziness or fainting).

Gluten Sensitivity/Intolerance:

Gluten intolerance and gluten sensitivity are terms highly disputed and difficult to distinguish, as opinions between scientists and physicians differ.

What we know is that it includes a spectrum of symptoms, disorders and effects. Those who suffer from gluten intolerance or sensitivity experience problems such as bloating, abdominal pain, diarrhea, constipation, irritable bowel syndrome, muscular disturbances, headaches, migraines, acne, fatigue, bone and joint pain.

OTHER BENEFITS OF GOING GLUTEN-FREE

Dr. William Davis wrote an extraordinary article in Life Extension Magazine, Oct. 2011. It is called *Wheat: The Unhealthy Whole Grain Book Excerpt: Wheat Belly*. It is worth reading, as it explains from a scientific perspective the issues related to wheat consumption and its impact on the body.

Increased Energy Levels:

It has been reported that people who consume too much gluten experience a lot of tiredness and weakness. Gluten-related fatigue can be disruptive and debilitating.

Researchers are still not entirely clear what causes fatigue in those with Celiac Disease or gluten-intolerance. But fatigue is recognized as one of the top symptoms. One speculation is that fatigue is caused by malnutrition or anemia.

Improved Digestion:

A gluten-free diet maintains and improves the digestive system. A lot of people who have undertaken a gluten-free lifestyle notice a mild to drastic change in terms of their digestion in a short period of time. They have said that there has been a noticeable improvement in bowel movements and a great reduction in indigestion. There is also a significant decrease in bloating and cramps, which is a definite plus for women.

Reduced Joint Inflammation:

A gluten-free diet also reduces inflammation in various tissues in the body. People who are highly sensitive and allergic to gluten usually experience episodes of pain in joints, muscles, and legs. People who also experience inflammation of the skin such as Dermatitis, Eczema, or Dermatitis Herpetiformis will reap some benefits from a gluten-free lifestyle, as well.

On the Dementia Diet my husband has noticed that he experiences less pain in his hips and knees.

Improved Blood-Sugar Levels:

Going gluten-free will help keep your blood sugar levels at bay. Food products with gluten are usually accompanied by significant sugar. So switching to a lifestyle made up of more single ingredients like fruits and vegetables and foods that do not contain gluten will help you to control your blood sugar and fat intake.

Beware of Processed Gluten-Free Packaged Foods:

According to a study by researchers at Dalhousie University in Halifax, Canada, published in the Canadian Journal of Dietetic Practice and Research in 2008, gluten-free products are a $4.2 billion dollar enterprise in the United States and $90-million in Canada.

This study also revealed that gluten-free products are 242% more expensive than their regular counterparts, and 455% pricier in some cases.

This is certainly true for me. I pay over $6.00 for a loaf of frozen gluten-free bread, but I eat so little of it, that it's worth the investment.

Gluten-free packaged food is a huge market. They are convenient, but many have more sugar, fat and calories added. Or the fiber has been removed. There is no need to go this route.

"Being gluten-free is a good thing, but eating gluten-free processed foods is not a good thing," says US cardiologist Dr. William Davis, author of the best-selling book Wheat Belly: Lose the Wheat, Lose the Weight and Find Your Path Back to Health. (CTVNews.ca)

Eating too much gluten-free processed food (what I call gluten-free junk food) like gluten-free cookies, cakes and processed food has a high glycemic load on your system. Just because it is gluten-free, doesn't mean it is healthy. Gluten-free cakes and cookies are still cakes and cookies! Vegetables, fruits, beans, nuts and seeds and lean animal protein are all gluten-free -- stick with those.

"We don't want to replace one problem with other problems," says Dr. Davis. "Foods that raise your blood sugar sky-high, make your tummy grow, give you hyper-tension, dementia, cancer and heart disease." (CTVNews.ca)

In an organic nutshell:

a) The wheat we consume today is not the same wheat consumed by our ancestors.
b) Today's wheat is believed to be troublesome for everyone.
c) Oats are gluten-free, but can be contaminated with gluten during processing. Make sure your oats are gluten-free.
d) A gluten-free diet reduces body and brain inflammation, fatigue and improves digestion and blood sugar levels.
e) Stay away from packaged gluten-free foods. They are processed and are usually high in fat and sugar.

Chapter 7: The Glycemic Index and Gluten-Free Grains, Legumes and Vegetables

The gluten-free diet requires the complete elimination of all wheat, rye and barley products. So, too, does the Dementia Diet.

Gluten-free replacements for cereals and baking mixes are often made up of a combination of cornstarch, potato starch, tapioca starch and/or white rice flour. The nutrient composition of these ingredients falls short in comparison to those provided by whole grains.

That's why it is important to incorporate gluten-free whole grains into your diet. Without whole grains, you can become deficient in important minerals, vitamins, fiber, calcium, and iron.

A study published in the American Journal of Clinical Nutrition underscores the importance of choosing whole grains such as brown rice rather than refined grains, i.e., white rice, to maintain a healthy body weight. In this Harvard Medical School / Brigham and Women's Hospital study, which collected data on over 74,000 female nurses aged thirty-eight to sixty-three years over a twelve year period, it revealed that women who consumed more whole grains were 49% less likely to gain weight compared to those eating foods made from refined grains.

Gluten-free whole grains can be low, medium and high on the glycemic index.

What is the glycemic index?

As explained earlier, the Glycemic Index (GI) is related to carbohydrates, which our body uses to make glucose, which acts as fuel.

When carbohydrates are consumed, the GI measures the speed of sugar entering the bloodstream. Every carbohydrate has a Glycemic Index. Some are low while others may be moderate or high.

The GI ranges from 0 to 100, and helps us understand how our body breaks down carbohydrates minus fiber.

Some foods cause quick and dramatic peaks (high glycemic foods) in blood glucose, while others do not (low to moderate glycemic foods). The lower the GI, the slower the effect of glucose on our blood sugar levels. One hundred equals pure glucose or sugar.

This is called the Glycemic Load (GL) and as stated earlier is probably more important than the GI as it takes into consideration how quickly a certain food converts to sugar (GI), as well as how much sugar a particular food contains. If a food is low in sugar it will have a low glycemic load.

Two foods can have the same glycemic index, yet produce different amounts of insulin. Or two foods could have the same glycemic load, but cause different insulin responses.

Inside the world of gluten-free, some flours, for example, have a lower glycemic index than others.

Turning high glycemic foods into slowly digested ones:

Jack and I only enjoy gluten-free pasta made from quinoa or corn flour. It's delicious. Rice flour and other versions of pasta like buckwheat taste either mushy or like cardboard to us. But corn has a higher GI index. To combat this GI index issue, I add soluble fibre or resistant starch foods (explained in next chapter) to the tomato sauce. Sometimes I'll add buckwheat. We love chunky tomato sauce! Soluble fiber and resistant starch slows digestion. This little trick helps to decrease the pasta's high glycemic impact on our blood sugar levels.

On the Dementia Diet you don't have to give up your favorite high-GI, gluten-free foods. Just eat them in moderation and balance them with resistant starch, soluble fiber, proteins, unsaturated fats (like MCT oil) and other low-GI complex carbohydrates. And be sure to only eat them occasionally and in smaller portions.

Let's get back to the glycemic index of gluten-free whole grains...

Grains should be stored for no longer than a year in a cool, dark place. Millet should be consumed within two to three months. Whole grain flours will last up to six months or in the freezer for up to a year.

When cooking whole grains, remember that they double or triple in size once cooked. For flavoring add broths, stocks, juice or milk in place of water. Before cooking grains, be sure to rinse them first. Bring the liquid to a boil and then reduce to simmer. You need not stir the grains. Once the grains absorb the liquid and are tender, remove them from the heat and let them sit for about 5 minutes.

Cook more than you need and store the extra cooked grains in the freezer.

In undertaking the gluten-free lifestyle, there are whole grains that support weight loss and others that sabotage it.

Here is a list of gluten-free grains and their general glycemic index:

Buckwheat (Low GI):

Despite its name, buckwheat is not wheat. In fact, it isn't a grain at all. It is a fruit seed of a plant related to rhubarb. These grain-like seeds have a unique triangular shape and are the same size as wheat kernels. Buckwheat can be ground into flour and substitute wheat, rye, barley and oats in recipes.

If you are embracing the Dementia Diet lifestyle, then you'll want to also embrace this fruit! It is fat free, low in calories, fills you up faster, controls blood sugar, facilitates proper digestion, builds lean muscle mass and suppresses the appetite. What more can you ask for in a seed?

Buckwheat contains a medicinal chemical that strengthens capillary walls and reduces haemorrhaging, lowering the risk of fatal strokes and heart attacks in people with high blood pressure and diabetes. It improves micro vascular integrity and circulation in diabetics, preventing nerve damage and loss of kidney function.

As a good source of magnesium, buckwheat helps to improve blood pressure by relaxing the blood vessels. Buckwheat's iron, magnesium, phosphorus, copper and manganese help to improve blood oxygenation. It contains high quality proteins, which remove the plaque forming triglycerides and low-density lipoproteins (LDL).

Buckwheat contains D-chiro-Inositol. This is a compound that is deficient in type 2 diabetic patients and is required for proper conduction of insulin for controlling and treating type 2 diabetes.

Because it is composed of cellulose, buckwheat removes toxins from the body, acting as a cleansing ingredient. And as an insoluble fiber, buckwheat helps to prevent gallstones. It speeds up the removal of food through the intestines, increases insulin sensitivity but lowers the secretion of bile acids and blood sugar.

A diet rich in buckwheat can also help reduce the risk of breast cancer. Its antioxidant properties are also beneficial for women during and after menopause, thus protecting against the risk of breast cancer and other forms of cancers related to hormones.

Buckwheat has an abundance of other health benefits, as well. It strengthens bones by facilitating the absorption of calcium. It contains tryptophan to influence our mood and helps to prevent depression and strengthens our immune system against flu and the common cold.

The secret to implementing buckwheat for weight loss is to eat it partially raw. When it is cooked buckwheat loses its nutrients and properties and its abilities to clean the body. When toasted, buckwheat is called Kasha. In Russia, Kasha is served with onions and brown gravy.

To Cook: There is a sweet spot for where your buckwheat will be tender enough to eat, but is not mushy. Bring 2 cups of water to a boil in a medium saucepan with some salt. Stir in 1 cup of buckwheat and bring back to a boil. Keep the lid off. Once the buckwheat starts to expand and all the visible water is absorbed, turn down the heat to low and place the lid on the pot. Leave the buckwheat to cook for another 5 to 15 minutes, depending on the consistency you desire. Check it regularly.

Quinoa (Low GI):

Quinoa has been a staple in the South American diet for centuries. It is a seed and a relative of spinach, kale and Swiss chard. As a super food, quinoa is low in calories and rich in dietary fiber and protein.

On the glycemic index, quinoa is as low as vegetables. Its dietary fiber binds to fat and cholesterol, filling you up quickly, causing your body to absorb less fat and cholesterol and reducing plaque build-up in arterial walls. This means quinoa helps to reduce the risk of heart disease and strokes. It is an excellent source of iron, calcium, magnesium, and B vitamins.

To Cook: To remove the bitter coating before cooking be sure to rinse quinoa several times in a fine-mesh strainer. Combine 1 cup of quinoa with 2 cups of water in a medium saucepan. Bring to a boil. Cover, reduce heat to low and simmer until quinoa is tender, about 15 minutes. When cooked, drain the quinoa for 15 minutes; otherwise your dish will be watery. Return quinoa to the hot pot. This allows it to dry out.

Quinoa is a great rice substitute.

Teff (Low GI):

For thousands of years teff has been a staple in the Ethiopian diet. It is an ancient North African cereal grass and super food! It is also the world's smallest grain and is 40% resistant starch, meaning that half the calories consumed cannot be absorbed.

Resistant starch foods like teff can help you lose weight if you use it as a substitute for pasta or add it to your pasta sauce. What's unique about teff is that it is packed with Vitamin C. (Grains are normally devoid of this vitamin.) Teff possess the eight essential amino acids a body needs to properly grow. Teff also helps manage blood sugar levels and triggers beneficial bowel movements.

It has a mild, nutty flavor and can be used to make polenta, cookies, breads, stews and so much more.

To Cook: Rinse teff under cold water. Add 1 cup of rinsed teff and 3 cups of water to a pot. Bring to a boil. Turn the heat to simmer, cover the pot and let cook for about 10 to 15 minutes. Turn off the heat, and let the teff sit for about 10 minutes. This allows the teff to absorb all the water. It should be sticky and nutty.

Wild Rice (Low GI):

Not far from our home is a Canadian aboriginal reserve called Curve Lake Reserve. Here wild rice is manufactured in small quantities and sold at our local farmer's market. This rice is absolutely delicious. You can smell the toasted grains while it's boiling in the pot.

Wild rice isn't really rice at all. It is the fresh water grass seed with twice the protein and fiber of brown rice, thus giving it a lower GI index. It is rich in antioxidants, possessing thirty times more than white rice, thus reducing bad cholesterol and the risk of cardiovascular disease. It's a good source of vitamins and minerals include Vitamins A, C and E, phosphorus, zinc and folate.

To cook wild rice, bring 3 cups of water to a boil and add 1 cup of rice. Reduce the heat and simmer on low for 40 to 45 minutes or just until kernels puff open. Uncover and fluff the rice with a fork. Drain off any excess liquid. This rice has a natural affinity to mushrooms. It can be served as a side dish or in soup, salad, pilaf, stuffing, casserole and pancakes.

Sorghum (Low GI):

Originating in Africa about 8000 years ago, sorghum is a cereal grain used in gluten-free cooking. Because it doesn't possess an inedible hull like other grains, sorghum is commonly eaten with all its outer layers, thereby providing your body with its nutrients. It is also grown from traditional hybrid seeds and so does not contain traits gained through biotechnology. It is non-transgenic (non-GMO). It is great for weight loss as sorghum digests more slowly with a lower glycemic index, and so sticks with you a bit longer than other flours or flour substitutes. It also helps to speed up the metabolism and at the same time supports it. Sorghum contains magnesium and copper, minerals that play an important role in food metabolizing. Packed with antioxidants, this cereal helps to reduce the risk of cancer and cardiovascular disease.

Sorghum can be substituted for wheat flour in a variety of recipes. It's neutral, sometimes sweet and is easily adaptable. It improves the texture of recipes.

To Cook: Rinse, drain and pick through sorghum. Combine 3 cups of water or stock with 1 cup of sorghum in a pot with a lid. Bring to a boil. Cover, reduce the heat to low and let simmer for about 50 to 60 minutes. Drain any excess water.

Brown Rice (Moderate GI):

Because of its high fiber, brown rice fills the stomach quickly. This generally leads to smaller meal portions, helping to inadvertently eat less.

Brown rice is considered one of the world's healthiest foods. It is a whole grain with its inedible outer hull removed, while still retaining its nutrient-rich bran and germ. (White rice is both milled and polished, removing the bran and germ along with all the other layer-rich nutrients).

Brown rice comes in short, medium and long lengths and in a whole bunch of different varieties with flavors and aromas. Some of the most popular varieties include: Long grain brown rice, with springy character, is well suited for casseroles and baked dishes. Medium grain brown rice is stickier and ideal for Spanish dishes like paellas. Short grain brown rice has creamy texture and can be used in risotto. Brown basmati rice is firm and has a dry consistency, ideal for biryanis and pilafs. Aromatic jasmine rice is moist and tender and good for Asian dishes and Kalijira rice grains are fast cooking and can substitute couscous-based dishes.

One cup of brown rice provides the body with 80% of its daily manganese requirement. Manganese is important to help synthesize fats. It is a good source of selenium, phosphorus, copper, magnesium, and niacin and fiber, fatty acids, amino acids and more. Due to its massive nutritional value, brown rice helps to prevent heart disease, cancer, diabetes, gallstones, asthma and rheumatoid arthritis.

To Cook: Rinse rice until the water runs clear. In a medium saucepan add 2 tablespoons of olive oil. Heat the oil, then add 1 cup of rice. This helps to build the flavor of the rice. Add 2.5 cups of water and a pinch of salt and bring to a boil. Reduce the heat to simmer, cover the pot and let simmer until the rice is tender, about 40 minutes. When the rice has finished cooking and the water has boiled off, let it rest with the lid on, for about 5 minutes.

Millet:

Originating in China, millet is a small-seeded grass, considered a cereal crop. Today it is revered in both India and in parts of Africa. Unfortunately, in North America it is primarily grown for birdseed.

Millet is highly underestimated and under-used in the kitchen. Considered an alkaline food with a moderate Glycemic Index, it is easily digested and has low simple sugars. Some of its vitamins and minerals include vitamin B3, copper, manganese, phosphorus and magnesium. This grain is high in fiber and so helps prevent gallstones and breast cancer.

Like all other grains, rinse millet under cold water before cooking to get rid of any dirt or debris. Add one-part millet to 2 parts water. Bring the water to a boil and reduce the heat to simmer. Cook millet for about 25 minutes or until the grain is fluffy like rice. It can be served as porridge, in bread, muffins, as a side dish, and in croquettes.

Amaranth (High GI):

It is not really a grain, but rather a seed belonging to the Amaranthaceae (pronounced am-a-ran-tha-see-a) family. This seed has a significant amount of the essential vitamins A, C, E, K, B5, and B6, folate, niacin and riboflavin. It is also rich in lysine (an amino acid) calcium, potassium, iron, copper, magnesium, phosphorus and manganese, protein, dietary fiber, and amino acids — all essential for a healthy body. Lysine in particular is believed to help reduce the risk of cancer and lower bad cholesterol. Amaranth is also great in boosting the immune system. It helps fight off certain diseases such as cardiovascular disease and hypertension.

Amaranth's moderately high content of oxalic acid inhibits much of the absorption of calcium and zinc. It should be avoided or eaten in moderation by those inflicted with gout, kidney disorders or rheumatoid arthritis.

While packed with vitamins and minerals, amaranth is high on the Glycemic Index, so eat it moderation and in small portions.

To Cook: 1 cup of amaranth to 3 cups of water. Bring to a boil, and then simmer for 25 minutes. The final consistency will be thick, like porridge. If you want to combine amaranth with another grain, substitute it with about ¼ of the other grain, then cook as you would for that grain.

Corn is a fruit:

Corn is a mysterious one, a fruit popularly known as a grain, and yet it is eaten as a vegetable. It is a staple in gluten-free breads, pasta and prepared foods and so I have included it here in this section on grains.

All varieties of corn – white, yellow, blue, purple and red – possess various antioxidants and phytonutrients. The variety of corn determines its content and type and level of phytonutrients. Colour plays an important role in the kinds of phytonutrients consumed. Yellow corn has carotenoids, while the blue variety has anthocyanin antioxidants, the same ones found in red wine.

Corn is also high in fiber, helping to reduce the risk of colon cancer and intestinal issues. It is also high in B-complex vitamins (B1, B5 and folic acid).

When eaten in moderation, corn has proven to be beneficial in controlling blood sugar in both type 1 and type 2 diabetes.

Keep in mind that while corn (as the fruit eaten like a vegetable) is beneficial on the Dementia Diet, high fructose corn syrup is sugar. Fructose goes right to the liver and triggers lipogenesis -- the production of triglycerides and cholesterol. This is a major cause of a condition known as fatty liver disease. The glucose in corn syrup triggers big spikes in insulin. The body disturbances from both the fructose and glucose increase the appetite, leading to weight gain, diabetes, heart disease and dementia!

Low Glycemic Legumes:

Legumes are a plant family made up of beans, peas, lentils, soybeans and peanuts. Yes peanuts!

Their defining characteristic is that they contain seedpods that split into two halves. Most are low on the glycemic index, are gluten-free and rich in nutrients. The ones dense in fiber include black, pinto, kidney, garbanzo, split peas, Lima beans and black-eyed peas.

Legumes are also part of the Mediterranean diet, which has been found to lower the risk of Alzheimer's and dementia. Legumes are low in fat and packed with antioxidants and minerals, such as calcium, copper, zinc, iron and potassium. Some of the essential vitamins in legumes include B vitamins and folic acid.

This list refers to dried beans and peas when boiled in water, along with their GI Index. Canned products tend to have a higher glycemic index.

Black-eyed peas 33-50
Butter beans average 31
Chick peas (garbanzo beans) 31-36 (canned 42)
Kidney beans 13-46, average 34
Kidney beans (canned 52)
Lentils 18-37
Lentils, canned 52
Navy beans (white beans, haricot) 30-39
Navy beans, pressure-cooked 29-59
Peas, dried, split 32
Pinto beans 39
Pinto beans, canned 45
Soybeans 15-20
Soybeans, canned 14

Low Glycemic Vegetables:

The list is arranged alphabetically. (Exact carb count depends on serving size.) Keep in mind that the fiber in vegetables can be subtracted from the total amount of carbohydrates.

Alfalfa Sprouts, Artichokes, Asparagus, Avocado;
Bamboo Shoots, Basil, Bok Choy, Broccoli, Brussels Sprouts;
Cabbage (or sauerkraut), Carrots, Cauliflower, Celery Root, Celery, Cilantro
Collards, Cucumbers (or pickles without added sugars);
Eggplant, Endive;
Fennel;
Green Beans, Green Bell Peppers;
Jalapeno Peppers, Jicama;
Kale;
Leeks, Lettuce;
Mustard Greens;
Nori;
Okra, Onions;
Parsley, Pumpkin;
Radicchio, Radishes, Red Bell Peppers, Rutabagas;
Scallions, Snap Peas, Snow Peas, Spaghetti Squash, Spinach, Summer Squash;
Tomatoes, Tomatillos, Turnips;
Water Chestnuts, Waxed Beans;
Zucchini

Glycemic Index of Starchy Vegetables

Beets 64
Carrots 16-92 average 47
Corn 37-62, average 53
Parsnips 97
Peas, green, fresh or frozen 39-54, average 48
Potato 56-111 - most averages usually given in high 80's
Potato, instant - 74-97, average 80

Rutabaga 72
Sweet potato - 44-78, average 61*

In an organic nut shell:

a) Eat lots of low glycemic, gluten-free whole grains.
b) Eat lots of low glycemic vegetables.
c) Eat lots of legumes.

Chapter 8: Healthy Starch! REALLY?

Eating in a way that balances your blood sugar, reduces inflammation and oxidative stress, and improves your liver detoxification is the key to preventing and reversing insulin resistance and diabetes and therefore Alzheimer's and dementia. Resistant starch should be part of your diet for this reason. There are 2 types of starches – digestible and resistant.

Unhealthy Digestible Starch:

As stated earlier in the section on diabetes and dementia...

Bread and pasta are examples of digestible starches. Digestible starches cause a rise in blood sugar, which causes a spike in insulin levels. Over time, the body cannot produce enough insulin, thus causing insulin resistance or metabolic syndrome. This leads to pre-diabetes and type 2 diabetes. People with type 2 diabetes have a lower level of cognitive function and are at higher risk for dementia. That's why it's important to eat bread and pasta occasionally, incorporating protein and fat, and to eat smaller portions.

Healthy Resistant Starch:

Resistant starch is different, in that it moves completely through the small intestine without being digested. As a result these starches act like soluble fiber. They help to lower fat intake because they have fewer calories than other starches. They assist in the fermentation of good bacteria in the gut that can affect our hormones, body fat, and glucose and glycemic index levels in a way that encourages a healthy body weight and even weight loss if desired. Resistant starch takes a longer time to digest. That means expanding as it soaks up fluids in your stomach stimulating satiety and giving you effective control over your appetite. Natural resistant starch foods also help diabetics manage their condition by decreasing glycemic response and increasing insulin sensitivity.

Research has shown that resistant starch foods have health benefits, such as:

- positively affecting our hormones
- aiding in weight loss
- *improving insulin resistance*
- *lowering insulin and glucose levels after meals*
- making more butyrate than other prebiotics
- lowering the risk of bowel cancer
- bolstering immune system
- improving gastrointestinal health
- improving kidney health

Here is a list of resistant starch foods to include in your Dementia Diet menu:

Green Bananas: (1 medium peeled, 4.7 g of resistant starch):

In North America we seem to only like ripe bananas. But green bananas are an integral part of other cultural menus, such as in the Caribbean and Jamaica. Green bananas contain inulin, a resistant starch that serves as a strong probiotic in the body, improving the health of gut flora as well as controlling blood sugar. I like to incorporate green bananas into bread. It's fabulous in shakes and frozen yogurt.

White Beans: (1/2-cup, prepared, 4.5 g):

White beans offer a double benefit for the gluten-free eater. They are high in resistant starch and are low in fat. Beans reduce blood sugar, and create the fatty acid butyrate, which burns fat faster. Studies have shown that butyrate improves mitochondrial function in your cells, leading to a decrease in fat. If you are concerned about gas, fret not. The more beans you eat, the more your body will build up the good bacteria to digest them. I love to puree white beans with garlic, fresh lemon juice, Parmigiano-Reggiano and freshly ground black pepper to taste. Spread the mixture on gluten-free rice crackers.

Lentils: (1/2-cup, 3.7 g):

Lentils are legumes, the seeds of plants whose botanical name is lens ensculenta. In North America we consume green or brown lentils. But they are also available in black, yellow, red and orange. Lentils readily absorb the flavors of the other ingredients in a dish and they have high nutritional value, as well as being a high resistant starch with no fat! Lentils are a good source of cholesterol lowering fiber and prevent the blood-sugar level from rising after a meal. While giving the body energy, lentils also help reduce the risk of coronary heart and cardiovascular disease. They are a good source of folate, copper, phosphorus, manganese, iron, protein, B1, zinc, potassium and vitamin B6.

Before cooking lentils spread them out and remove any stones. Then wash them thoroughly. Place them in boiling water for 20 to 30 minutes, depending on their end use. Often this legume gets overlooked or type-casted in the roll as a soup and stew ingredient. But lentils can be used in making burgers, omelets, dips, chili, sloppy Joes, vegetarian Moussaka, tacos, Indian Mango Dal, risotto, salads and even cabbage rolls.

Yams: (1/2-cup, cooked, 2.5 g):

I probably eat more sweet potatoes than yams. But yams are a resistant starch and certainly more enticing from this perspective. Yams are different than sweet potatoes. The flesh inside a sweet potato is orange. The flesh inside a yam is white to purple. Yam is the starchier and drier distant cousin of sweet potato. It originated in Africa where 95 percent of the crops are still grown. The rough scaly skin ranges from off-white to dark brown. Yams are low in fat and are a good source of vitamin C, B6, thiamin, manganese, copper and potassium. It is a healthy complex carbohydrate that helps the digestive tract and aids in decreasing the risk of obesity, heart disease and several forms of cancer.

We tend to stick to one yam dish – candied yams. But yams can be incorporated into the bean burrito, stews and soups, kebabs, gluten-free breads, mashed with potatoes, garlic and Parmesan and more.

Chickpeas: (1/2-cup, prepared, 2.0 g):

I think my husband and I survive on chickpea dip called hummus with gluten-free tortilla chips. It certainly wards off hunger pains until dinner. In a food processer or blender combine 2 cups of canned chickpeas (drained and rinsed) with 3 tablespoons of tahini, 2 cloves of garlic, 2 tablespoons of lemon juice, ¼ cup of coconut or olive oil, and kosher salt and black pepper to taste. This Middle Eastern legume can also be used in salads, burgers, and soups. Chickpeas can also be pureed with yogurt and cumin and served as a dip. Besides being a resistant starch, chickpeas boost your energy, stabilize blood sugar levels and are high in protein and have a low glycemic index. They reduce bad cholesterol, aiding in the reduction of the risk of heart disease.

Green peas: (1/2-cup, prepared, 2.0 g):

Green peas are not as powerful a resistant starch as green bananas, but they are packed with other nutrition that's hard to beat.

Green peas, in the legume family, are a nutritionally loaded addition to soups, salads, as a side dish, or in stir-fries and noodle dishes, to name but a few. They contain important fat-soluble nutrients like beta-carotene, vitamin E, Omega 6 fatty acid and linoleic acid. Some other green pea health benefits include anti-aging, a strong immune system and high energy. These benefits come from their flavonoids (catechin and epicatechin), carotenoids (alpha and beta-carotene), phenolic acids (ferulic and caffeic acids) and polyphenols (coumestrol).

Due to their strong anti-inflammatory properties, vitamins C and E and Omega 3 fatty acids, green peas help to prevent wrinkles, Alzheimer's, arthritis, bronchitis, and candida. They are high in fiber and so regulate the blood sugar level, aid in the reversal of insulin resistance (type 2 diabetes) and improve bowel health. With an abundance of vitamin B1 and folate, B2, B3, and B6, vitamin K (anchors calcium), green peas aid in the prevention of heart disease and osteoporosis as well.

When purchasing fresh green peas look for pods that are firm and smooth. They should have a medium green color and are flat. If the color is dark, yellow, whitish or specked with gray, avoid them.

Brown Rice: (½ cup, cooked, 1.6 g):

Brown Rice is covered in Chapter 2.

Kidney Beans: (1/2-cup, prepared, 1.4 g):

When combined with rice, this legume provides an excellent source of protein – without the high calories and fat of red meat! In fact, one cup of kidney beans provides 15.3 grams of protein, 30% of one's daily requirement.

Like most beans, kidneys are also an excellent source of cholesterol lowering fiber. Hypoglycemic and diabetic friendly, these beans help to stabilize blood sugar levels after meals.

One of the best benefits of kidneys is that they are high in 'molybdenum.' Molybdenum is a trace mineral and an important part of the enzyme called sulfite oxidase, which is responsible for detoxifying sulfites in the body.

One cup of cooked kidney beans supplies about 177.0% of our molybdenum daily requirement. I checked my multivitamin. It contains eight mcg of this trace mineral. For the human being, seventy-five mcg of molybdenum is a daily requirement. So, kidney beans are now a part of our weekly gluten-free food repertoire.

Molybdenum is believed to help to protect the stomach and esophagus against cancers, aids in the absorption of iron and so helps to prevent anemia, as well as tooth decay. Molybdenum also aids in the metabolizing of fats and carbohydrates. (Other than kidney beans, other foods high in molybdenum are meats, buckwheat, barley, wheat germ, lima beans, sunflower seeds and dark green leafy vegetables.)

Most importantly, kidney beans are high in soluble and insoluble fiber. Soluble fiber produces a gel-like substance that increases stool bulk and therefore helps to prevent constipation.

When buying kidney beans at bulk food stores, look closely to ensure they are not cracked.

To prepare dried kidneys quickly and for culinary greatness, rinse the beans under cool water. Place them in a pot on a burner with just enough water to cover. Bring the water to a boil and then let the beans simmer for 2 minutes. Remove the pan from the heat. Let the beans stand in their liquid for two hours. Remove the beans from this liquid. Discard the liquid. Rinse the beans under cool water again. Put them into a clean pot. Add 3 cups of water to every 1 cup of beans. Bring the water to a boil. Reduce the heat to simmer. Let the kidneys cook for another 1.5 to 2 hours until soft and done.

Kidney beans are part of Chili con Carne. But they can also be incorporated into pasta salad or a salad of fresh greens with cilantro and walnuts. Kidney beans are also part of the classic bean salad and will act as a dense and tasty binding agent in vegetarian burgers.

Quinoa: (1/2-cup, cooked, 1.0 g):

Quinoa is a super food and we really should incorporate it more into our diet. We certainly do not eat enough of it. Quinoa originated in South America and has been a staple in the South American diet for centuries. More than a grain it is a seed relative of spinach, kale and Swiss chard. As a super food, it is low in calories and rich in dietary fiber and protein.

Quinoa is also low on the glycemic index, as low as vegetables. And due to its fiber content, quinoa makes you feel full much faster. Its dietary fiber binds to fat and cholesterol, which causes your body to absorb less fat and cholesterol. The fiber found in quinoa also reduces the plaque build-up along your arterial walls, which reduces your risk of heart disease and stroke. Quinoa contains high quality protein and has a protein profile similar to cow's milk. It is an excellent source of iron, calcium, magnesium, B Vitamins and riboflavin.

To Cook: Rinse it well. There is a bitter coating on the tiny seed that needs to be rinsed away. When rinsing it, use a fine-mesh strainer. Combine 1 cup of quinoa with 2 cups of water in a medium saucepan. Bring to a boil. Cover, reduce heat to low and simmer until quinoa is tender, about 15 minutes. When cooked, drain the quinoa for 15 minutes; otherwise your dish will be watery. Return quinoa to the hot pot. This allows it to dry out.

Potatoes: (1/2-cup, cooked/mashed 0.6 to 0.8 g):

Jack and I love potatoes in gluten-free Sheppard's Pie (with ground chicken, beans and lentils) and in soups and stews with peas and carrots and other soluble fiber ingredients. We always incorporate potatoes with fat and protein and soluble fiber to help slow the digestion of this high glycemic food. Despite the bad press, potatoes are a resistant starch packed with nutrients. Potato is rich in immune-boosting vitamin C and B, potassium, magnesium and iron. It contains a blood pressure lowering chemical called kukoamines, which the Chinese use in making teas for lowering blood pressure. With sixty different kinds of phytochemicals and vitamins, the potato reduces the risk of cardiovascular disease and bad LDL-cholesterol and helps to keep arteries clear.

Did you know that one potato serves as twelve percent of your daily-recommended dose of fiber? They improve bowel health and support healthy digestion. Rich in vitamin B6, this tuber helps to reduce stress. Stress reduction aids in weight loss.

In an organic nut shell:

a) Foods with resistant starch aid in preventing insulin resistance, diabetes and therefore dementia.
b) Foods with resistant starch act like soluble fiber, have fewer calories, help to lower fat intake and take longer to digest, thus keeping blood sugar levels from spiking.
c) Choose dishes or make recipes possessing high resistant starch, such as green bananas, white beans and lentils.

Chapter 9: Fat is Back

Both healthy fat and bad fat effect brain shrinkage in the Alzheimer's brain. Fat is one of the body's building blocks. The average person is made up of between 15% to 30% fat. What we know is that the higher the quality of the fat, the better the body and brain uses that fat to build cell walls and therefore function more efficiently.

In fact scientific studies have shown that those with the largest brains and highest test scores had blood that contained high levels of vitamins B, C, D and E and also the seafood type of Omega-3 fatty acids.

You'll know if your body is not getting enough fat. Some of the warning signs include:

- dry skin
- soft and brittle nails
- stiff joints
- tiny bumps on the backs of your arms

There are different types of dietary fats. They are:

- Trans Fat
- Saturated
- Mostly Polyunsaturated
- Mostly Monounsaturated

FATS AND DEMENTIA:

Upon first visiting Mr. Levy, he asked me to immediately stop giving Jack the supplement called Omega 3-6-9. He told us that Omega 6 and Omega 9 causes inflammation of the body and the brain. He put Jack on a sublingual Omega 3 –D3 supplement consisting of 3020 mg of Omega 3 fatty acids in one teaspoon. This is broken down into 1900 mg of EPA and 900 mg of DHA and 220 mg of other Omega 3 fatty acids. This one teaspoon also includes 1000 IU's of vitamin D3.

Omega 3:

Omega 3 is covered more extensively in Chapter 11. In fact scientific studies have shown that those with the largest brains and highest test scores had blood that contained high levels of vitamins B, C, D and E and also the seafood type of Omega-3 fatty acids.

Research also shows that Omega 3 may seriously influence dementia risk. Its benefits include increase blood flow to the heart and blood vessels; anti-inflammatory effects; and support and protection of nerve cell membranes.

Suffice to say that inflammation can be a key factor in the development of many diseases, including dementia and heart disease. Omega 3 fatty acids are converted into inflammatory proteins, but at a much slower rate. The body's natural mechanisms of breaking down inflammatory mediators occur before inflammation has a chance to take place. We know that Omega 3's lower the risk of heart disease and stroke, increase concentration and help those suffering from inflammatory conditions, such as rheumatoid arthritis. They also help prevent Alzheimer's, according to a new American study.

Flaxseed oil is primarily Omega 3 fatty acids and contains both stearic and palmitic saturated fatty acids. By percentage of total fats, flaxseed oil is 58% Omega 3s, 14% Omega-6s, and 19% monounsaturated fats, 4% stearic acid and 5% palmitic acid. It is extremely sensitive to oxygen, light and temperature. Keep it stored in a cool, dark place, like the wine cellar! It should be used as a drizzle or in vinaigrette or sauce. Never use flaxseed oil for cooking. When heated its flavor changes to paint-thinner.

Omega 6:

Studies have found that 'overdosing' on oils rich in Omega 6 (safflower or sunflower oil) could possibly double the risk of developing dementia. One of the reasons is that Omega 6 is pro-inflammatory and Omega 3 is anti-inflammatory. Omega 6 is pro-inflammatory because it is broken down by the body and converted into prostaglandins and other inflammatory proteins. In fact, medications such as ibuprofen and naproxen work by blocking the formation of these same inflammatory proteins. Oils high in Omega 6 include corn oil, but also peanut oil, grape seed oil, cotton seed, safflower and sunflower oils. Store bought dressings and pre-made mayonnaise is loaded in Omega 6 fats.

Omega 9:

Omega 9 fats are known as non-essential. The reason is that the body can synthesize them from the foods we eat. We need not depend on a supplement to obtain Omega 9. The main Omega 9 is oleic acid, found in olive oil, canola oil, peanut oil and sunflower oil. It also has an inflammatory effect on the body and brain, according to Jack's physician.

Trans Fats:

An investigation at Portland's Oregon Health and Science University, lead by Dr. Gene Bowman, looked at the effect of trans fats on the brain. They studied the blood samples and MRI brain scan results of 104 seniors with an average age of 87 years. The study revealed that those with higher levels of trans fats in their blood had smaller brains and scored lower on thinking and memory tests. Removing trans fats from your diet can improve over all brain health, memory and thinking.

Trans fats can also induce inflammation by damaging the cells in the lining of blood vessels.

Over fifteen years ago I became aware of Dr. Udo Erasmus, M.D. and his booked entitled 'Fats that Heal Fats that Kill'. This is a fantastic book that discusses research on common and the lesser-known oils with therapeutic potential, such as flax, hemp, olive, fish, evening primrose, borage, black currant and even snake oil! In his book, Dr. Erasmus also exposes the manufacturing processes that turn healing fats into killing fats. They are called trans fats. He explains the effects of these damaged fats on our bodies.

If there were such a thing as evil in the culinary world, trans fat would be the devil. Trans fats are more like plastic than food, proven to raise LDL cholesterol (bad) and lower your HDL cholesterol (good), thus elevating the blood cholesterol level and therefore contributing toward heart disease.

As it cannot be overstated, much evidence supports the link between an elevated blood cholesterol level, type 2 diabetes and the development of Alzheimer's and dementia. In experiments, animals fed high-fat and high-cholesterol diets exhibited impaired learning and memory performance compared to those under a controlled diet. In fact one study consisting of 444 Finnish men revealed that an elevated blood cholesterol level in midlife was associated with three times the risk of developing Alzheimer's later in life.

We know that the brain is made up of 60% fat. Trans fats replace healthy fats like Omega 3 fatty acid (DHA) in the brain's cell membranes, and therefore affects the brain's ability to properly function. As a result cellular communication suffers, blood flow is restricted, the cells degenerate, the brain shrinks and memory and cognition are affected, thus potentially increasing the risk of dementia.

Its other aliases are trans-fatty acids, partially hydrogenated vegetable or soybean oil. The hydrogenation process was developed in the early 1900's. Vegetable shortening was one of the first products to be made from this ingredient. At one time trans fats were considered a healthy alternative to saturated fat. By the late 1950's, the American Heart Association began recommending the reduction of saturated fats. Trans fats made its way into processed foods because it was and remains a preservative. It extends product shelf life. Fried foods, frozen pizza, cakes, cookies, margarine and spreads, pie, ready-made cake frostings and coffee creamers all contain trans fat. Even whipped cream can contain this devil-of-an-ingredient. Thought to be healthier, hydrogenated vegetable oil became the ingredient of choice for frying, sautéing and baking by both chefs and home cooks alike. While many restaurants have eliminated trans fats in their establishments, others have not.

In 2013 the FDA banned the use of trans fat in foods due to its detrimental health effects. Trans fat is slowly being phased out. Until it is completely eliminated from products, it is still important for you to read labels to hunt for it. I say "hunt" because the nutritional chart on a food label may read "0 g trans fat". This doesn't necessarily mean the product is trans fat free. It can still contain up to half a gram of trans fat per serving. Instead, read the ingredient list. Make sure the product is free of "partially hydrogenated oils."

SATURATED FATS:

Not all saturated fats are bad.

Saturated fats are solid at room temperature. For decades we've been told that saturated fat leads to cardiovascular disease. New studies, research and evidence suggests otherwise. A review in the American Journal of Clinical Nutrition showed an analysis from data pooled together from twenty-one studies made up of 350,000 people, about 11,000 with cardiovascular disease. After fourteen years, the study concluded that there is no relationship between the intake of saturated fat and the incidence of heart disease or stroke. This doesn't mean one should gorge on animal fat. Remember beef particularly can be loaded with hormones and antibiotics. Poultry can also have an overload of antibiotics. Your animal proteins should be grass fed and organic.

If your recipes call for ingredients with saturated fat, choose healthier versions. If your recipe calls for butter, use butter. Just head to the health food store and choose raw, organic butter or instead use butter spread (made up of butter and either olive or vegetable oil). While butter is a type of saturated fat, it's also loaded with nutrition. Butter is rich in Vitamin A, lauric acid, lecithin, anti-oxidants, Vitamins E and K, selenium, linoleic acid, Vitamin D, to name a few. Simply said, butter treats fungal infections, is essential for cholesterol metabolism, protects against free radical damage, fights cancer, builds muscles, boosts one's immunity and protects against tooth decay. Shall I go on? So why give up butter? Just choose healthy versions of saturated fat and eat them in moderation or on special occasions.

Palm Kernel Oil (89% Saturated):

Palm kernel oil comes from the nut of the African palm tree. It is composed of fatty triglycerides. It is cholesterol-free and contains vitamin K. Vitamin K is an essential fat-soluble vitamin that is important for blood coagulation. It is used in the making of supermarket products like margarine, ice cream, chocolate, shortening and creamers. Doughnuts, ramen noodles, potato chips, French fries and other fast foods are made with palm kernel oil. Remember this oil is still high in saturated fat, which can add weight gain if not consumed in moderation. Today this product is used in heart healthy butter spreads (not margarine), ice cream, chocolate, shortenings and creamers.

MCT Oils (Palm Kernel and Coconut Oils):

Palm kernel oil and coconut oil (covered in the next chapter) are saturated fats high in desirable medium-chain triglycerides or MCTs. MCTs are considered gold to the starved brain.

Both oils contain lauric acid with its antibacterial, anti-viral and most importantly *anti-inflammatory* properties!

MCT oil is also tasteless. It is a fabulous ingredient to be incorporated into soups and salad dressings, sauces, stir-fries, casseroles, pasta dishes and drizzles. Endless are the uses for MCT oil. And you never get tired of its taste because it is tasteless.

Coconut oil contains about 60% MCTs. But MCT oil contains 100% MCTs! Medium Chain fatty acids have tremendous health benefits.

The fatty acids in MCT's are as follows:

Caproic Acid (C6)
Caprylic Acid (C8 about 6% in coconut oil)
Capric Acid (C10 about 9% in coconut oil)
Lauric Acid (C12 and 50% of coconut oil)

C6, C8 and C10 are found in coconut oil and in other sources such as goat's milk. The word "Capra" means goat.

Caproic Acid, (C6): is found in coconut oil to a smaller extent. It tastes terrible, can cause a burning sensation in the throat and can cause gastric issues.
Caprylic Acid (C8): has powerful anti-microbial properties to provide good gut health. This is an important fatty acid for the brain because of its ability to provide good gut health.

In simple terms a healthy gut ensures a healthy blood brain barrier (BBB). It is now believe that the breakdown of the BBB may be involved in several brain diseases, including Alzheimer's, epilepsy, multiple sclerosis, etc.

One of this fatty acid's other best features is its ability to fight a yeast fungus in your gut called candida. New research reveals that the fungus Candida makes the exact same type of amyloid plaque that has been found in Alzheimer's brain.

In doing extensive bloods tests on Jack, Dr. Levy found that he was infected with a high level of Candida in his body. Dr. Levy introduced Caprylic acid into his dietary plan to kill the Candida. We both continue to take Caprylic acid (an oil) on a daily basis. It is our daily source of MCT oil.

Did you know that you need about 18 tablespoons of coconut oil to obtain just one tablespoon of Caprylic acid?

Capric Acid (C10): is the second shortest form of MCT. It is also rare. It is slower to turn into energy, but more affordable than Caprylic Acid.

MOSTLY MONOUNSATURATED FATS:

Monounsaturated fats are liquid at room temperature but solidify in the refrigerator. They are believed to help reduce bad cholesterol levels in the blood and therefore lower the risk of heart disease and strokes. Monounsaturated fats also help to speed up your basal metabolic rate (BMR). This is the rate at which calories are burned when you're in a state of rest. The calories are used to sustain basic functions such as cell repair, maintain body internal temperature and pump blood throughout the cells.

Macadamia Nut (85% Monounsaturated):

Indigenous to Australia, the Macadamia nut is now grown commercially in Hawaii, California and Florida. It is the highest in monounsaturated oil, higher than flax seed or olive oil. The oil is also perfectly balanced in Omega 3 and Omega 6. For this reason I use is sparingly. It is not only heart healthy, but contains a high amount of oleic acid, a type of monounsaturated fat that lowers the LDL cholesterol from the blood and is believe to preserve brain health by keeping your blood pressure low and preventing strokes. Macadamia nuts also possess a fatty acid known as palmitoleic acid, an important component of myelin, the fatty layer that insulates and protects nerve cells in the brain.

Olive Oil (75% Monounsaturated):

Olive oil is packed with monounsaturated fat and antioxidants. This heart-healthy fat protects blood vessels throughout the body, including the brain. Olive oil is at the heart of the Mediterranean diet, which is believed to help prevent

Alzheimer's and other dementia. It is no secret that Alzheimer's and dementia is lower in countries with populations consuming the Mediterranean diet and olive oil.

Did you know that there is more Italian olive oil distributed throughout the world than there are Italian olives growing! How is this possible? We, the public, are purposefully misled about olive oil authenticity and quality. Many olive oils are not pure. Many are blended with other oils, such as canola. People (like me) use these inferior blends, thinking they're doing good things for their body. How do you find pure olive oil? Look for the family's name on the bottle. Also, the product should be "made in Italy" NOT imported from or bottled in Italy. The address of the estate should be present on the bottle, as well. And most importantly, there MUST be a Lot #. Every pure bottle that leaves Italy (sealed) is given a Lot #.

Jack and I have been using olive oil as a body moisturizer. Pure extra virgin olive oil is the best thing for one's skin. Use it right on your skin. This protects the skin from all the bad ultra violet rays that cause skin cancer. The best sunscreen. It you rub olive oil on your skin and it sits on top and is greasy, it's not pure. It is no doubt blended with other bi-products. PURE virgin olive oil have small molecules that allow the pores to quickly absorb it. Pure olive oil also reduces wrinkles if you mix some with a little lemon juice and use it on your face at night. For your hair, after shampooing, mix some olive oil, lemon juice and an egg yolk, and a little bit of beer together. Rub this mixture into your hair and leave it on for 5 minutes. Rinse.

The olive oil experts (who must train as diligently as wine sommeliers) say that you should not put ANYTHING on your skin that you would not put into your mouth. Everything that goes onto the skin is absorbed into the brain within ten seconds. Olive oil is the most effective and safest product for the skin, for aging, for sun protection, and for aiding in the prevention of skin cancer.

"Pure virgin olive oil" also does the following...

- reduce LDL cholesterol
- reduce arterial occlusion
- reduce angina and myocardial infarction
- reduce blood glucose and triglyceride levels
- increase bile secretion for improved digestion
- aid in liver detoxification
- increase vitamin A, D and E absorption
- heal sores
- reduce gallstones
- improve membrane development, cell formation and cell differentiation

Avocado Oil (63% Monounsaturated):

Jack and I consume avocados on a regular basis. We love avocados in sandwiches and gluten-free pasta salad. I also make gluten-free avocado and key lime pie and add this fruit to our homemade frozen berry yogurts.

Unlike other fruits, avocado is mostly made up of 85% healthy fat rather than carbohydrate. Some of its nutrients include Omega 3, vitamin K, folate, vitamin C, potassium, vitamins B5 and B6 and vitamin E. The avocado has smaller amounts of magnesium, manganese, copper, iron, zinc, phosphorous, vitamin A and B1 (thiamine), B2 (riboflavin) and B3 (niacin).

As a monounsaturated fatty acid, it has also been shown to:

- ease arthritic pain, due to anti-inflammatory properties from its carotenoids and phytosterols and polyhydroxylated fatty alcohols (PFA's)
- lower blood pressure, due to its combination of Omega 3's, oleic acid and potassium
- increase blood flow, due to its high vitamin K content, thus decreasing the risk of stroke which can lead to vascular dementia
- help lower our risk of heart disease

- prevent insulin resistance which can lead to type 2 diabetes and dementia
- prevent the formation of brain tangles, due to its high Folate
- support the digestive tract to increase absorption of fat-soluble nutrients, due to its Oleic acid

Canola Oil (55% Monounsaturated):

This is our Canadian oil. The name represents "Can" for Canada and "ola" for oil. It is now produced in Canada and mostly in the Pacific Northwest. It is high in mono-saturated fat and has a good balance of Omega 3 and Omega 6. (Because of its Omega 6, I use this oil sparingly.)

The canola plant is part of the same botanical family as cabbage, broccoli and cauliflower. It is the Brassica family. The oil comes from its crushed seeds. The canola seed is about 45% oil. The oil itself has the least amount of saturated fat of any cooking oil. In fact it has half the saturated fat of olive and soybean oil. Because of its neutral flavor, canola oil has an important place in the culinary world. For example, it can be used in vinaigrettes when you want other flavors (besides the oil) to shine through. If making a tomato and avocado salad with a tangerine vinaigrette, I use canola oil because of its neutral taste. It allows only the tangerine flavor to predominate and therefore adds only weight and stick-ability to the vinaigrette. I made up that word, stick-ability. It means the oil sticks to the greens. For friends I recently made baked salmon with fresh herbs and caramelized lemons and drizzled the fish in a pink grapefruit hollandaise sauce. Rather than using olive oil, which adds a distinctive taste, I chose canola to let the pink grapefruit flavor take center stage.

Red Palm Oil (40% Monounsaturated Fat):

Red palm oil comes from the bright red flesh of the fruit of the palm tree, albeit a different variety of tree than what produces palm kernel oil. Both oils have completely different vitamin and mineral properties. Red palm oil contains high levels of vitamins A and E, as well as ten carotenes including alpha-, beta-, and gammy-carotenes, sterols, and antioxidants, phenolic acids and flavonoids. Because its fatty acids are stable, it has a smoke point of 302F and so can be used as a cooking oil. Store this oil in the wine cellar.

Red palm oil is believe to help reduce the risk of the following diseases:

- Alzheimer's
- Arterial thrombosis
- Atherosclerosis
- Blood clotting
- Cancer
- Cataracts
- Cognitive impairment
- Macular degeneration
- High blood pressure
- High cholesterol levels
- Vitamin A deficiency

MOSTLY POLYUNSATURATED FATS:

Polyunsaturated fats are liquid at room temperature and remain this way in the refrigerator.

Grape Seed (71% Polyunsaturated Fat):

Do not overdose on grape seed oil. Use it sparingly, as it is high in Omega 6, potentially causing inflammation in the body and brain. I use it sparingly.

A European staple for generations, grape seed oil has finally come to the mainstream supermarket shelves. It is light green in colour and lightly flavored and loaded in polyphenols. Studies suggest that grape seed oil can lower bad cholesterol (LDL) levels and raise levels of the good kind (HDL). There is also evidence that it may aid in healing arterial walls. Research has also shown that grape seed extract helps to reduce cognitive impairment and brain degeneration in mice and stop small clusters of A-beta protein that poison brain cells and memory loss. This research shows significant promise that grape seed oil extract could work toward preventing Alzheimer's disease. Grape seed oil has a fairly high smoking point, so it is effective for pan frying and baking. It also makes for a tasty base ingredient for vinaigrette.

Camelina (57% Polyunsaturated Fat):

This oil comes from the Camelina Sativa seed, also referred to as 'false flax.' It was harvested and used for centuries as an oilseed crop for lighting lamps in Europe and North America. It is largely unsaturated (90%) and high in Omega 3 fatty acids (39%) and Omega 6 fatty acids (18%). While it contains some Omega 6, it is prized for its richness in ALA, EPA, DHA, and vitamin E, supplements that support the prevention and slowing of dementia due to its high Omega 3 (anti-inflammatory and anti-arthritic properties).

In Canada we have a well-known camelina oil producer called Three Farmers in Saskatchewan (www.threefarmers.ca). This producer follows the Farm to Fork movement focused on connecting consumers with all stages of food production - from growing to harvesting to processing to consuming. At Three

Farmers, they strive to provide this personal connection between their farmers and customers by implementing traceability. This refers to the fact that every step in the food production process is transparent. By entering the code found on every bottle of Three Farmers camelina oil into their website, the complete history of your bottle of oil can be discovered, from the moment the seed was sown to which the farmers planted it.

Three Farmers takes a holistic approach to sustainable agriculture, engaging only zero tillage farming techniques, which preserves the soil structure and nutrients. They also employ inter-cropping, which is the practice of growing two or more crops in the same field at one time. Thus, each crop can give the other what it requires in terms of nutrients, all the while maintaining the integrity of the soil. This is also a non GMO product and their oils are available in a variety of tasty flavors like Roasted Garlic and Chili and Roasted Onion and Basil.

The oil has a nutty taste and high heat point and so also has its place in the culinary world. It can be used for sautéing, frying, baking, and in vinaigrettes, drizzles, etc.

In an organic nut shell:

a) The higher the quality of the oil (fat) that you eat, the better your brain function.
b) Consume coconut oil and MCT oil on a daily basis.
c) If you have dementia avoid foods high in Omega 6 and Omega 9 and avoid Omega 6 and Omega 9 supplements. They contribute to inflammation of the body and of the brain.
d) Consume foods high in Omega 3. Omega 3 breaks down inflammation, lowers the risk of heart disease and stroke and increases brain function and concentration.
e) Stay away from foods with trans fats.
f) Eat foods incorporating monounsaturated fats, such as olive oil and avocado oil and macadamia nuts.
g) Eat organic, grass fed proteins (which possess healthy saturated fat.) Grass fed beef is high in Omega 3.

Chapter 10: The Power of Peanut Butter Brain Bars

I created the Peanut Butter Brain Bar as a way for Jack to ingest a minimum of 3 teaspoons of coconut oil per day. As a saturated fat, the oil is solid at room temperature. This makes it challenging to find ways for Jack to take the oil on a regular basis. I tried putting the oil in homemade ice cream. It made the ice cream lumpy. He didn't like tasting it with hot water and lemon each morning either. It felt like just another chore for him, on top of his morning medications and vitamins. I tried several recipes, aiming to find one that enticed Jack to willingly take the coconut oil each day.

Jack loves peanut butter and coconut and, of course, everything sweet. So I decided to make the Peanut Butter Brain Bars as a kind of treat or dessert, knowing he would look forward to eating them. I didn't call them by this name right away.

If you and/or your loved one is allergic to peanuts, use almond butter, which is available is most supermarkets and can be made fresh at many health food stores. If you are allergic to nuts altogether, use pumpkin seed butter instead of peanut, almond or cashew butter and use sunflower or sesame seeds instead of walnuts.

The name 'Peanut Butter Brain Bars' evolved in a way for him to remember them. With the bars I can be assured that Jack remembers to eat at least one each day without my nagging him. He never eats more than 2 per day because they are so decadent and rich.

I purchased a colourful container that fits into my freezer for the bars. I set them in layers divided by parchment paper. He has no trouble pulling the container out and returning it to the freezer. We keep the bars frozen as this makes them crunchier. They can also be kept in the refrigerator.

The Peanut Butter Brain Bars have proved to be an enormous success with Jack. The bar's effect works immediately. This is a two-inch square consisting of peanut butter, coconut oil, unsweetened shredded coconut and a thin layer of bittersweet chocolate. It's sweetened with stevia and/or coconut palm sugar.

I have noticed a significant difference in Jack's cognitive function once he has had his bar. In the winter Jack puts on his coat so I can take him to Starbucks for his morning coffee and workout at the gym. Without taking his brain bar, Jack struggles with doing up the zipper of his winter coat. It can take him between three to ten minutes to figure out the zipper and sometimes he gives up altogether. He just resorts to asking me to zip up the coat for him. And Jack hates asking me to do this as he is committed to remaining independent.

Within 10 minutes of taking the brain bar, Jack can zip up his coat in under a minute. This is just one specific function that is immediately improved through his consumption of coconut oil on a regular basis.

My family has also noticed a huge improvement in his communication skills since starting on the brain bars. He can take part in normal conversations without forgetting what he wants to say. The benefits are incredible.

I believe the Peanut Butter Brain Bars are the most important part of Jack's Dementia Diet. He has eased into the routine of eating two bars per day, one in the morning and one for dessert after dinner.

The bars are also popular amongst family and friends. Some of my girlfriends eat them because they are so delicious and because the bars support healthy brain function. Everyone wants a healthy brain. The recipe is at the end of this chapter.

Coconut Oil (90% Saturated Fat):

For thousands of years coconut oil has been a healing agent. Western science is just catching on to the power of this super food.

Coconut oil is saturated fat but don't be alarmed. Not all saturated fat is bad.

A Cleveland dentist named Dr. Weston Price (1870-1948) is renowned for discovering the origins of tooth decay. He believed that the human diet was the source of society's health, vitality and well-being. In the 1930's, he traveled through the South Pacific, researching traditional cultural foods in an attempt to gage effects of diet on teeth and health. Dr. Price realized that those societies with diets high in coconut were healthy and slim, despite the oil's concentration of saturated fat.

Then came the 1950's and all saturated fat became unfairly vilified. A pioneer investigator named Ansel Keyes proclaimed that heart disease was related to hydrogenated vegetable oil. This newfound proclamation made the food-grade oil industry upset. As the story goes, as a defence they created a marketing campaign to vilify another oil on the market in an aim to take the focus off their own product -- hydrogenated vegetable oil. Saturated fat became the villain.

In the 80's researchers studied two Polynesian populations. Coconut was a primary source of caloric intake. The American Journal of Clinical Nutrition published studies that showed that both these populations possessed positive vascular health.

Today the truth has been unveiled. Hydrogenated vegetable oil (trans fat) is a primary factor contributing to heart disease and Alzheimer's. Avoid it at all cost. We also know that organic, grass-fed proteins (with saturated fat) are healthful when consumed in moderation and coconut oil (another saturated fat) is a super food. We have since learned that lauric acid (in coconut oil's saturated fat) increases good HDL cholesterol. Coconut oil also improves digestion, boosts thyroid function, boosts metabolism, gives us energy and endurance, and improves our overall health of skin and hair.

Coconut oil is brain food, acting like an alternative fuel (energy source) in the insulin-deficient or starved Alzheimer's brain.

Dr. Mary Newport, M.D is author of the book, "Alzheimer's Disease: What If There Was a Cure?" I highly recommend this book. In 2000 Dr. Newport began to see signs of progressive Alzheimer's in her husband Steve at age 53. He started on Alzheimer's drugs, but the disease continued to worsen. She researched ways to slow its progression and discovered that some brain cells may have a difficult time using glucose, the brain's major energy source. Without this fuel, brain neurons die. She knew that an alternative energy source for brain cells is fat, since the brain is made up of 60 to 70% fat.

Coconut oil is 90% saturated fat, 66% of its fat being medium-chain triglycerides (MCT's). These fats bypass the bile and go directly to the liver, converting the oil to ketones. The liver releases the ketones immediately into the bloodstream. Once in the bloodstream the ketones move to the brain and are used as fuel. The brain treats the ketones like a carbohydrate (sugar) rather than like fat. This is why the ingestion of coconut oil (or MCT oil) has immediate effect on the brain, especially with persons with dementia and Alzheimer's. This is why Jack is able to perform functions so quickly after eating a Peanut Butter Brain Bar. Research is being conducted to see if ketone bodies actually help to restore nerve function in the brain.

Dr. Newport started her husband on two tablespoons per day of coconut oil and began cooking with it throughout the rest of the day. She discovered that after 60 days Steve was more alert in the morning, showed more animation in his face, and seemed to have more personality. Steve told her that his taking the coconut oil felt like a fog had lifted from his brain and that he had gotten his life back. He continued to return to himself over the weeks and months to follow.

(As an aside, the body also converts the MCT's to monolaurin. Monolaurin is a chemical with antiviral and antibacterial properties. These properties help the body prevent colds, flu, swine flu, herpes, shingles and other infections. Monolaurin is also believed to treat chronic fatigue syndrome.)

A recent University of Oxford study supports Dr. Newport's theory that ketones play an important role in brain health. However, the study does suggest that the benefits from coconut oil may be temporary. But for those of us who are caregivers, any benefits, short or long term, are everyday mini-miracles. And if this means having Jack eat Peanut Butter Brain Bars for the rest of his life then that's the way it's going to be.

Let me add that I do not advocate taking Peanut Butter Brain Bars and eliminating traditional dementia medications. I advocate an approach that brings together allopathic medicines and naturopathic remedies, under the supervision of your physician. In our case it is under Dr. Levy's supervision.

Organic, cold pressed, non-hydrogenated, virgin coconut oil is key. Any part of the coconut, except for the water, has sufficient levels of the oil. Coconut oil can be found in the milk, meat, grated or in the oil itself. Coconut capsules possess only 1 gram of coconut oil. Yet there are fourteen grams of oil in every tablespoon. So, fourteen capsules are required to get the same amount of oil as in one tablespoon.

Coconut oil is worth ingesting whether you're the person with dementia or a caregiver. Add coconut oil to your diet slowly and increase slowly to avoid diarrhoea and other intestinal issues. Start with one teaspoon taken with meals two to three times per day. Once gastro intestinal issues stop, increase the amount by one teaspoon with every meal, totalling between four to nine tablespoons per day. It's also a great natural remedy for constipation!

If you're making the bars, start with half of a bar for the first couple of weeks.

The Peanut Butter Brain bars are integral to Jack's cognition and functions. That's because they contain three important brain-healthy ingredients – peanut butter, coconut oil and shredded coconut and walnuts.

Peanut Butter:

When developing the Peanut Butter Brain Bars, I started with peanut butter as the next primary ingredient because Jack absolutely loves it. It's also healthy. We purchase organic freshly ground peanut butter at the health food store and I add a little Stevia.

A serving of peanut butter has 3 mg of the powerful antioxidant vitamin E, 49 mg of bone-building magnesium, 208 mg of muscle-friendly potassium, and 0.17 mg of immunity-boosting vitamin B6. Research shows that eating peanuts can decrease your risk of heart disease, diabetes, and other chronic health conditions. One study published in the *Journal of the American Medical Association* found that consuming 1-ounce of nuts or peanut butter (about 2 tablespoons) at least 5 days a week can lower the risk of developing diabetes by almost 30%.

So what does this have to do with dementia and Alzheimer's?

Well, we know that diabetes is the 7th leading cause of death in the US. Among older adults with diabetes, there is an association between low blood sugar (hypoglycemia) and dementia, says researchers at the University of California, San Francisco, in a new study published in the Journal of the American Medical Association. This can create a dangerous spiral in which a hypoglycemic event caused by diabetes can lead to mental deterioration and vice versa.

What doctors, researchers and scientists now know is that Type 2 diabetes is a major risk factor for Alzheimer's, vascular dementia and other types of dementia because cardiovascular problems associated with diabetes are also associated with dementia. These problems are:

- Obesity
- Heart disease
- Circulation problems
- High cholesterol
- High blood pressure

Alzheimer's is now being called type 3 diabetes. Recent studies suggest that the Alzheimer's brain is now believed to be in a diabetic state, partly due to the decrease of or insensitivity to insulin. Insulin helps blood cells take up glucose, which means that for diabetics, getting glucose to the brain can be challenging. A brain starved of energy can develop neurological problems like dementia and Alzheimer's disease.

Simply said, what is good for the heart is also good for the brain. Peanut butter is good for both. Eaten regularly and in moderation, organic, sugar-free peanut butter decreases the risk of heart disease, diabetes and therefore Alzheimer's and other dementia.

Walnuts:

The brain has 100 billion nerve cells or neurons. They communicate together and exist within networks. Some networks control thinking and learning, while others allow us to hear, smell, and see.

In the Alzheimer's brain, two abnormal structures called plaques (known as beta-amyloids pronounced as BAY-tuh AM-uh-loids) and tangles (called tau and rhymes with 'wow') damage nerve cells. The Alzheimer's brain appears to have more of these plaques and tangles than the average brain. Plaques and tangles are believed to play a role in blocking communication between the nerve cells, thus disrupting the processes that allow the cells to survive. While not yet scientifically proven, it is believed that the death of the nerve cells in the Alzheimer's brain contributes to personality changes, memory failure and other symptoms.

Omega-3 fatty acids, found in proteins like chicken and fish and also in nuts are believed to help lower the blood levels of the plaque (the beta-amyloids.) Research has found that the more Omega 3 a person takes per day, the lower their blood beta-amyloid levels. Consuming 1 gram of Omega 3 per day is associated with 20% to 30% lower blood beta-amyloid levels.

Walnuts are now believed to help prevent and even slow Alzheimer's and other types of dementia.

The Peanut Butter Brain Bars contain 2 cups of organic, unsalted walnuts. By eating 2 brain bars per day you are getting between 1 to 2 ounces of walnuts per day, containing 2.5 grams of Omega 3 fatty acids.

Along with benefiting the brain, walnuts help lower bad cholesterol and increase HDL or good cholesterol levels in the blood. Thus adding walnuts to your diet might help prevent coronary artery disease and strokes.

Walnuts are also a rich source of anti-oxidants known to have potential health effects against cancer, aging, inflammation, and neurological diseases. The hormone melatonin in walnuts also helps to induce and regulate sleep.

Peanut Butter Brain Bars:
Makes 23 (2-inch x 1-inch) bars

Jack eats one of these squares 2 times per day. They are low in sugar and high in coconut oil. He gets at least 3 teaspoons of coconut oil per day by consuming the squares.

Chocolate Base:

¼ cup organic, virgin coconut oil
¼ cup stevia (powder)*
6 (1 oz.) bitter chocolate squares (no sugar)

Coconut Mixture:

2 1/2 -cups organic sugar-free peanut butter**
¼ cup of coconut palm sugar
1-cup organic, virgin coconut oil
3-cups unsweetened shredded coconut
2-cups of unsalted walnut pieces

*Stevia comes in various forms, such as powder or liquid extract. When purchasing it, read the label to ensure the product is not filled with fillers. Avoid liquids with alcohols. With powder forms it should only say "Stevia." Trustworthy brands include NuNaturals and SweetLeaf.

**Sugarless, fresh organic peanut butter is available at a health food store. Add peanuts if you like. If you are allergic to peanuts, use almond butter.

Coat a 9 x 12 inch cookie sheet with parchment paper. Set aside.

In a Teflon coated sauté pan add coconut oil. Heat on low until melted. Add one bitter chocolate square at a time stirring with a rubber spatula constantly until all are melted. Add stevia, stirring constantly.

Pour melted chocolate on parchment paper and using rubber spatula smooth out to cover entire cookie sheet in a rectangle shape, making sure it is even and making a thin coat. Set in the freezer to harden.

In a food processor or blender add peanut butter, coconut palm sugar and coconut oil. Blend until creamy. Add shredded coconut. Coarsely blend into a coarse meal.

Transfer mixture to a bowl. Fold in walnuts. Remove chocolate base from freezer. Pour peanut butter mixture onto the chocolate and smooth over entire surface, making sure all the chocolate is coated. Make sure the mixture is evenly spread. Transfer back to the freezer for at least 2 hours.

Remove from the freezer and cut the slab into 2-inch x 1-inch squares.

Transfer squares to a container. Separating layers with parchment paper. Seal and put back into the freezer or refrigerator.

In an organic nutshell:

a) What is good for the heart is good for the brain.
b) A brain with Alzheimer's is now believed to be in a diabetic state. Alzheimer's is called type 3 Diabetes.
c) Coconut oil is high in medium-chain triglycerides, which have an immediate and positive effect on the brain.
d) Oils with MCT's also have monolaurin, which is anti-viral and anti-bacterial, thus warding off colds, flus, shingles and herpes.
e) Natural, organic peanut butter (sugarless) is good for the heart and good for the brain. It decreases the risk of diabetes and heart disease.
f) Walnuts are now believed to help prevent and even slow Alzheimer's and other types of dementia.
g) Eat peanut butter brain bars!

Chapter 11: Organic Proteins

The Dementia Diet advocates the eating of low glycemic fruits and vegetables, legumes, low-glycemic gluten-free and wheat-free grains, seeds and nuts. I also support the idea of eating dairy, fish, seafood, poultry and meats in moderation and on occassion, as long as the products are local and organic and the animals are grass-fed and treated humanely. Increasing research and studies show that the use of herbicides, fungicides and pesticides used in producing our food sources, is detrimental to our health.

Many new studies have found an increase in cognitive, behavioral and psychomotor dysfunction in individuals who were chronically exposed to pesticides and herbicides. It is not surprising that Vietnam veterans exposed to the herbicide called Agent Orange (which released the poison dioxin) are now in their senior years suffering from a whole array of diseases. The effects of this toxic herbicide has also negatively and deeply impacted the Vietnamese people and their country. Jack served three tours in Vietnam and was directly exposed to Agent Orange. Since he does not suffer from heart disease or diabetes and Alzheimer's is not part of his family genetics, we believe Jack's Agent Orange exposure may be the cause of his Alzheimer's. However, while not diabetic, Jack was addicted to sugar.

Published in the US National Library of Medicine National Institutes of Health, an abstract entitled 'Linking Pesticide Exposure and Dementia: What is the Evidence,' the authors state,

"Evidence from recent studies shows a possible association between chronic pesticide exposure and an increased prevalence of dementia, including Alzheimer's disease (AD) dementia. At the cellular and molecular level, the mechanism of action of many classes of pesticides suggests that these compounds could be, at least partly, accountable for the neurodegeneration accompanying AD and other dementias."

In an article published on the National Center for Health Research, dated April 14th, 2014 by Celeste Chen, she states, *"Over the next 40 years, the number of people in the world with Alzheimer's Disease, the most common form of dementia, is expected to triple. Because Alzheimer's strikes as people get older, the U.S. is expecting a big increase in this brain-wasting disease as baby boomers become seniors."*

Chen goes on to say that pesticides kill insects by attacking their nervous systems, and herbicides wipe out some plants but not others. Pesticides and herbicides, she believes, are increasingly being linked to diseases that attack our nervous systems and brains.

Chen says, *"Several studies have shown that individuals regularly exposed to pesticides and herbicides are more likely to develop Parkinson's disease (PD) which makes it difficult for people to control their movements and can cause emotional changes. Now, there is reason to believe that pesticide exposure can also increase a person's chances of developing Alzheimer's disease."*

Published research has shown a link between Alzheimer's and DDT, an ingredient used in many pesticides of the 1970's. DDT (dichlorodiphenyltrichloroethane) was banned in the U.S. in 1972, but people continue to come into contact with this dangerous pesticide by buying imported foods or by living in agricultural areas exposed to DDT.

Eat Fresh, Local and Organic:

One of the best ways to ensure products are free from herbicides, pesticides and fungicides is to eat organic and local when possible. Visit your local farms. I'm fortunate to be living in the heart of farm country where I can obtain local, fresh and organic products from our farmers and from our local, Saturday farmer's market. Small organic and sustainable farmers care about their impact on soil life and fertility, water systems and conservation, air quality and the sustainability of the local and big picture eco-system.

106

If you live in a metropolis then following this philosophy may be more difficult. However, you can Google, "Organic farms in (type in your city)." From here you can find farms closest to your home. Look at the websites of these farms to find out where their products are being sold within your city. Take a day trip and visit the farms.

I don't trust organic labeling on products in large scale production. Not all organic designations are legitimate. If you cannot buy from your local farms, talk to your health food supermarket purveyors and ask them to educate you on the companies with integrity who are producing 'true' organic products.

Nowadays supermarkets are carrying more local, fresh and organic products.

Beef:

I have pernicious anemia and so require sufficient doses of vitamin B-12 through food, vitamins and shots. Once in a while I crave beef. The fact is beef contains high quality protein and nutrients like Creatine and Carnosine, which are important for our muscles and brain.

We have a hefty beef farming industry in our community in Ontario, Canada. We also have very cold winters. Around the world there is much controversy over this term called 'grass-fed.' In our community cows are generally fed grass in the summer and finished on corn before processing. However, we also have a few organic farms. A local organic beef farmer feeds his cattle summer grass and in winter the cattle consume hay and legumes. The legumes are grown in the field with the grass and so are mixed when the hay is harvested and wrapped. (Finishing is a term used to describe the time that the cattle are fattened before processing).

I learned that cattle finished on corn and/or grain and given hormones can have a daily weight gain of up to three pounds. Finishing on corn gives the beef more fat marbling. Cattle finished on hay and legumes are generally smaller animals that gain about one pound in weight per day.

As a food writer aiming to please my guests when entertaining, I've always advocated for cattle finished on corn because this method provides the beef with more marbling, and therefore more fat, and therefore more flavor. And my adage has always been, "Where there's no fat, there's no flavor."

I love marbling! But since implementing the Dementia Diet I've embraced and implemented grass-fed beef into our diet. The cuts have little marbling and possess a deeper color of red. Dr. Mordy Levy advocates the consumption of organic, grass-fed beef on occasion and in moderation. Also medical research has linked the consumption of excessive animal fat to inflammation.

Every country has its own ideas and regulations about cattle feeding. I was told by this organic farmer that in Canada we have no organization advocating for organic, grass-fed cattle.

In the United States, cattle graze on grass for the first six months to a year of their lives, but then are finished at a feedlot. The cattle spend anywhere from 60 to 200 days at the feedlot where they are fed a concentrated combination of corn, soy, grains, supplements, as well as hormones and antibiotics. Those in this industry may refer to this as a 'balanced ration for optimum weight.'

During the 200 days at a feedlot the cattle gain as much as 400 pounds. If a cow can gain three pounds of fat per day and you multiply this by 200 days, it's easy to understand how this much weight can be acquired over 200 days. Once the cattle are fattened to their 'finished weight' they are transported to the slaughterhouse.

In my opinion, this occurs as inhumane.

According to the American Grassfed Beef Association, "an animal's nutrient profile can significantly change in that time. During those months of grain finishing, levels of important nutrients like Conjugated linoleic acid (CLA) and Omega-3 fatty acids decrease dramatically in the animal's tissues."

Research has now shown that CLA is a potent ally for combating cancers of the breast, colorectal, lung, skin and stomach.

This is an important point when you are considering the Dementia Diet. The more I can provide Jack with natural forms of Omega 3's and CLA, the better the health of his brain. On the Dementia Diet my commitment has moved from marbling to getting as much nutrients as possible out of the beef for our brain health.

I personally believe that the way cows are treated and fed has an effect on the nutritional value of the beef. Many scientists agree. (By the same token many cattle farmers and scientists disagree.) Everyone is entitled to their opinion.

As it was explained to me, cows naturally eat grass. This affects their digestive track, PH levels and the fatty acid composition of the meat.

According to an article by Dr. Rekha Mankad, M.D. on the Mayo Clinic website, "grass-fed beef may have some heart-health benefits that other types of beef don't have." Dr. Mankad goes on to say that grass-fed beef may have less total fat, more Omega-3 fatty acids, more conjugated linoleic acid (a type of fat that is believed to reduce heart disease and cancer risks), and more antioxidant vitamins, such as vitamin E and others.

There are three main types of saturated fat found in red meat. They are: stearic acid, palmitic acid, and mystristic acid. Grass-fed beef are believed to be consistently higher in proportions of stearic acid, which does not raise blood cholesterol levels.

If at all possible, buy beef directly from the farmer where you can witness first-hand how the animals live and are treated.

For Jack and I our commitment has changed to brain health rather than momentary culinary satisfaction. In our city we have a 'meatery' (fancy word for butcher shop), that produces their own line of grass-fed organic beef. The cuts are deep red and devoid of marbling. The finished products are absolutely delicious.

Fish and Seafood:

Did you know that the more Omega 3 fats you eat, the easier it is for the body to cool itself? A cool body is less inflamed. I've stressed throughout this book that inflammation leads to chronic diseases of the body and brain.

When Jack was diagnosed with Alzheimer's I soon learned about the links between Omega 3 fatty acids and an increase of brain volume (Alzheimer's shrinks the brain) later in life and its power to potentially ward off dementia altogether. The brain is 60% fat, the largest portion of which is an Omega 3 called docosahexaenoicacid (DHA). Your brain requires DHA to spark communication between cells. Feeding the brain with DHA boosts cognition, learning and memory.

A 3-ounce serving of salmon provides 1.9 grams of Omega 3 fatty acids. Herring is just as rich in Omega 3's. Tuna has slightly less. A 3-ounce portion of tuna provides 1.5 grams of Omega 3's. Anchovies and sardines contain 1.2 grams in a 3-ounce portion. Other fatty fish with Omega 3 fatty acids include mackerel, trout, and halibut.

Whether it is farm raised or wild, fish in general, is best to be consumed in moderation. A joint research effort between Biodiversity Research Institute and the International POPs

Elimination Network revealed that 84% of all fish on the planet are contaminated with unsafe amounts of mercury. In an article called *Mercury Contamination in Fish Expected to Rise in Coming Decades*, author Danielle Elliot of CBS News states, *"Mercury pollution from power plants in China and India is making its way into fish in waters near Hawaii, according to new research."*

In this article Elliot goes on to say that mercury produced by the coal-burning power plants in these northern Pacific countries travels thousands of miles through the air before rainfall deposits it on the ocean floor near Hawaii.

According to the Centers for Disease Control and Prevention in Atlanta, the negative effects of mercury poisoning include permanent kidney and brain damage. Effects on brain functioning can result in a list of issues, such as irritability, tremors, vision changes, hearing and memory problems.

Fish that feed at deeper levels of the ocean, such as swordfish, have higher mercury concentrations than those that feed in waters near the surface. Mahi-mahi and Yellowfin tuna are examples of high mercury fish. Other examples are mackerel, orange roughy, and shark. Fish with the lowest levels of mercury include sardines, anchovies, haddock, salmon, sole, tilapia, shrimp, crab and oysters, to name a few.

There are many Omega 3 supplement options and products from which to choose to ensure you are getting a daily sufficient level. As mentioned earlier, Jack and I take a pharmaceutical grade whole food sublingual Omega 3 plus Vitamin D3 supplement.

It is suggested that we should not eat fish more than once per month due to the potential of ingesting mercury and other toxic contaminants.

Farmed salmon are fed ground-up small fish that tend to have high concentrations of PCBs. Approximately 60% of all salmon consumed in the United States come from farms. PCBs are considered highly toxic, leading to cancer and fetal brain impairment.

I am a fan of our Canadian icon and scientist David Suzuki. He is committed to preserving and cleaning up our planet's oceans and educating and supporting responsible fishing and farming practices.

To learn more about eating the right kinds of fish and seafood visit his website or iPhone app called www.davidsuzuki.org

Poultry:

Remember an organic label does not mean the birds were treated humanely and allowed to run freely outdoors. Choose farms or companies that you know slaughter the chickens before they require antibiotics, living in clean conditions, are not over-crowded and can roam freely outdoors for a few seasons each year.

We have a local organic chicken farm in our community called Yorkshire Valley Farms. The chickens are fed a proprietary non-GMO, all-grain feed mix made up of organic corn, soy, and wheat. The grains are free of synthetic fertilizers, herbicides and pesticides. The farm refrains from adding animal by-products to the feed. The chickens are not treated with hormones or antibiotics. The company advocates that these organic practices reduce bird stress and encourage their own immune systems to keep them healthy. As a result the birds tend to be smaller and more expensive.

But this is the choice you make if you choose to follow the Dementia Diet. I have moved to purchasing Yorkshire Valley Farm chickens when shopping at my local supermarket. They are delicious chickens!

When dining out following an organic diet is almost impossible. So, Jack and I eat at home on a more regular basis, eating out less often.

Antibiotics and Hormones:

In North America hormones and antibiotics are used in food production. These additives help animals grow and increase lean tissue and reduced fat and reduce the animals' risk of illnesses and disease. These additives are used to produce healthier animals at a lower cost to the consumer.

In Canada growth hormones are given to beef cattle. Antibiotics are used in poultry, pork and farmed fish. Antibiotics can also be sprayed on fruit and given to honey bees. Be sure to investigate the regulations in your country.

Much controversy exists as to whether antibiotics and hormones are passed on to humans when they consume dairy and protein.

The safest approach is to follow these guidelines:

- choose local and organic grass-fed beef
- eat beef, eggs and diary in moderation
- choose organic free range poultry
- choose organic eggs
- choose wild fish and seafood
- wash all vegetables and fruits for at least thirty seconds under running tap water to minimize the intake of antibiotics

In an organic nutshell:

a) New research links pesticides and herbicides to the destruction of nerve systems and can cause dementia.
b) Too much animal fat can cause inflammation in the body and brain.
c) Organic, grass-fed beef is high in Omega 3 which increases brain volume.

d) Organic, grass-fed beef is high in CLA, which decreases the risk of heart disease and certain cancers.
e) Choose local and organic grass-fed beef.
f) Eat beef, eggs and diary in moderation.
g) Choose organic free range poultry.
h) Choose organic eggs.
i) Choose wild fish and seafood.
j) Eat fish and seafood in moderation.
k) Take an Omega 3 supplement.
l) Wash all vegetables and fruits for at least thirty seconds under running tap water to minimize the intake of antibiotics.

Chapter 12: Brain Vitamins and Minerals

When we first published this book many family, friends and readers asked us for brand recommendations for vitamins, supplements and dementia diet friendly foods. To respond to the numerous requests, we made our favorite brands available at:

www.dementiadietshop.com

At the moment there appears to be "insufficient" evidence within mainstream allopathic medicine, research, and studies to confirm that vitamin and mineral supplementation can slow or reverse the progression of dementia.

I have my own perspective on this matter. I've been a part of and have watched Jack's returns, his mini-miracles. I can speak from firsthand knowledge that the 7 Dementia Diet principles work.

Within this illusive medical community are highly-trained and respected individuals – well known neurologists, cardiologists, researchers, physicians and specialists to name but a few – who wholeheartedly believe that a healthy diet and vitamin/mineral supplementation will not only prevent, but also slow dementia progression. Dr. Levy, our functional medicine physician, also resides in this camp.

Making sure you are meeting your daily requirements of vitamins and minerals is important to everyone, whether you're the caregiver or the person with dementia. Daily requirements ensure that your body, in general, is functioning properly, that your energy level is high and you have the ability to fight off disease and infection.

Simply said, we all need sufficient levels of vitamins and minerals to enjoy a healthy quality of life. A healthy quality of life goes a long way in allowing the body to remain active and the mind positive.

Studies are also showing great promise to substantiate this perspective. For example, a new study was conducted to look at the effect of vitamin E and memantine on functional decline in Alzheimer's disease. The study, conducted at fourteen Veterans Affairs medical centers, assessed the effect of the vitamin alone or with memantine on functional decline in 613 patients (97% men). The study revealed that for patients with mild to moderate Alzheimer's, 2000 IU of vitamin E daily slows functional decline. The person with Alzheimer's showed returns in both bathing and dressing himself. These functional returns to oneself reduced the caregiver's burden on average of up to two hours per day. As a full-time caregiver I am excited by the results of this study!

(As an aside I have spoken at great lengths about Jack's mind, body and spirit returns. I have also personally noticed that my vitamin regime has made me mentally stronger and provided me with far more energy. I feel more positive and hopeful. That is not to say that my life is free of stress or free of long nights with no sleep. I still must battle adversities. However, I'm now rising at 5am with astounding alertness rather than dragging my butt out of bed at 7am. I'm up early even when I've had a restless night due to stress.)

As stated, our vitamin regimes were individually designed and are closely monitored by Dr. Levy. I stress that it's vital that you consult with all your healthcare providers regarding the potential pros and cons of vitamin supplementation for both the caregiver and person with dementia. Make sure that the supplements you take will not interfere or adversely interact with your medications. Dementia therapies, pharmaceutical or natural therapies should always be used under the direct supervision of your medical physician. I stress this point emphatically!

> "The Good physician treats the diseases; the great physician treats the patient who has the disease."
> - Sir William Osler, one of the first professors at Jack Hopkins University School of Medicine and Physician-in-Chief.

In Judith DeCava's book called, "The Real Truth about Vitamins and Antioxidants," she defines a vitamin as, "a complex mechanism...of functional, interrelated, interdependent components. A vitamin consists of, not only the organic nutrient(s) identified as the vitamin, but also enzymes, coenzymes, antioxidants and trace element activators."

She goes on to say that a vitamin complex is not simply an individual chemical or several chemicals. It must contain all factors that make up the vitamin in its entirety. Just like a car is not four tires, nor a wheel, nor an engine, but rather it is a "car" when all parts are complete and working together.

Vitamins are not created equally. Every country handles their vitamin supplement industry and quality standards differently. The bioavailability of vitamin supplements also vary from one product to the next. Bioavailability refers to the degree to which a nutrient becomes available to the target tissue after it has been administered.

Supplement standards vary from unacceptable to outstanding. Many manufacturers do not employ qualified PhD health researchers. Supplement formulations may not be based on good medical and scientific research either. In fact, most multivitamins and minerals don't contain the essential ingredients for optimal health nor do they possess the most beneficial ratio of ingredients. Many products are not tested and are not pure.

A new U.S. study lead by Erin LeBlanc, an endocrinologist with Kaiser Permanente Center for Health Research in Portland, Oregon (released in February, 2014) found a huge variation in the potency of vitamin D supplements manufactured by different companies. The study also revealed the grand discrepancy in pill potency from the same bottle. The supplements ranged from 9% to 140% of the amount listed on the label.

Added chemicals and fillers can be cork by-products, chemical FD&C dyes, sodium benzoate, dextrose, ethycellulose, and propyleneglycol to name but a few. These products are legal, but provide no nutritional value. If a supplement is not manufactured properly it may not work and over time could cause side effects.

When it comes to supplements there are also two boot camps. One side believes that vitamins can be synthesized in high concentrates known as synthetic. Most supplement manufacturers follow this perspective, the majority of which are pharmaceutical companies. While synthetic these supplements might also be labeled as 'natural', even if they derive from sugar.

The other boot camp believes that vitamins and minerals are complex and their parts are interdependent and therefore should not be separated. They are referred to as 'whole food vitamins' because they come entirely from whole foods.

Vitamin C is a perfect example. Vitamin C is often referred to as ascorbic acid. This is the case if the vitamin is synthetic. Synthetic vitamin C is ascorbic acid manufactured from super-refined corn sugar. And this may be sugar from genetically modified corn (GMO). Add to this that ascorbic acid has such a strong effect on the body that it will leech out its other necessary cofactors from the body in order to be utilized by the body. This puts stress on the body.

Ascorbic acid is also only the outer skin of vitamin C, much like the skin of a grapefruit. True vitamin C is gentler on the body.

In the United States there are three grades of raw materials used in products with the difference being of quality and purity. They are:

Pharmaceutical grade – meets pharmaceutical standards
Food Grade – meets standards set for human consumption
Feed Grade – meets standards set for animal consumption

United States Pharmacopeia (USP):

USP is a scientific, non-profit organization that establishes federally recognized standards for the quality of drugs, dietary supplements, and foods. They help manufacturers, suppliers, and regulators safeguard the dietary supplement industry by providing documentary standards and reference materials for determining ingredient identity, strength, quality and purity. USP provides third-party, independent assurance to manufacturers and the consumer that the quality and purity of the raw materials utilized are of pharmaceutical grade. The USP guarantees a certain standard of excellence. Products bearing this symbol are sold only through physicians and selected pharmacies. When choosing supplements look for the USP label.

In Canada (my country) vitamins and minerals must have a Drug Information Number (DIN). While this is not a guarantee of purity or quality, the number indicates that the Canadian government has at least 'looked' at the list of ingredients in the product.

Vitamins and minerals are regulated as a sub-set of drugs and governed by the Natural Health Products Regulations. These regulations stipulate that the manufacturers must employ qualified staff who are responsible for assuring product quality before the products are released for sale. Manufacturers are required to provide detailed information about quality as part of their product license applications. Complaints are investigated by Health Canada. The consistency of active ingredients in each batch of pills is also an issue in Canada.

Despite the country in which you live, your best assurance in getting quality supplements is to read the label. Look for:

- supplements made from organic whole food sources

- food sources that are GMO free
- pharmaceutical grade products
- an indication on the bottle that says 'this product is laboratory tested and its potency is guaranteed'
- an expiration date

Vitamin Regime:

Our vitamin regime consists of some liquid vitamin supplements that are absorbed through the mucous membranes of the mouth via sublingual liquid. Others come in capsule form. It's important to consult with your physician on specific dosages of each vitamin. Your individual regime should be designed accordingly. You are metabolically unique. You absorb some nutrients better than others and you may burn through certain vitamins more quickly.

All vitamins and minerals should be taken with food. The reason is that food slows down the transit time through the small intestine, which is where all vitamins and minerals are absorbed. A longer time in the intestine creates more opportunity for absorption.

Jack's Vitamin/Supplement Regime:

Dr. Levy put Jack and I on a daily vitamin/supplement regime consisting of the following:

- Vitamin B 1, 6 and 12 (sublingual)
- Omega-D3 Liquid
- Vitamin D3
- Mito-Matrix Advanced Antioxidant
- High Count, Multi-Strain Acidophilus and Bifidus
- Cogni-Q (PQQ + CoQ10)
- Vitamin E
- Multi vitamin
- Coconut oil or MCT oil (caprylic acid)
- Bioavailable curcumin (turmeric)

I choose not to give you the specific dosages, because I do not want to encourage you to take dosages into your own hands if you are a caregiver or if you have been diagnosed with dementia and are on medication. See your medical physician or naturopathic doctor or, like us, your functional medicine physician first.

WATER SOLUBLE VITAMINS:

B Complex:

An Optima team from the Oxford Project conducted a study about the effects of Vitamin B on Alzheimer's and dementia and to investigate memory and ageing. The results of the study were pleasantly surprising. The study showed that vitamins B6 and B12 combined with folic acid slowed atrophy of gray matter in brain areas affected by Alzheimer's. Brain shrinkage and the shrinkage of brain gray matter is responsible for mild cognitive impairment. This impairment can lead to dementia.

Half of the volunteers took a daily tablet containing levels of the B vitamins folate, B6, and B12 well above the recommended daily amount. The other half received a placebo. After two years in the study, the Optima research team measured the rate at which the participants' brains had shrunk. They discovered that in those participants taking the vitamin supplements, brain shrinkage slowed by 30%. In some cases brain shrinkage slowed more than 50%.

Working together B-complex vitamins breakdown carbohydrates into glucose to provide the body with energy, as well as breaking down fats and proteins. This group of vitamins also keeps our muscles toned, intestinal tract healthy and our skin, hair and eyes looking younger!

The B-complex vitamins consist of vitamins B1, B2, B3, B5, B6, B7, B9 and B12.

Vitamin B1 is thiamine and gives us nerve and muscle function and aids in our digestion. Milk, potatoes, sweet corn, liver and beans are all rich in thiamine.

Riboflavin is vitamin B2 and found naturally in asparagus, popcorn, bananas, milk, yogurt, meat, eggs, fish, leafy green vegetables, legumes, tomatoes, mushrooms and almonds, to name but a few. This vitamin helps to give us healthy skin, mouth and eyes and promotes energy production and antioxidant protection.

Vitamin B3 is also called niacin and is known for helping to eliminate depression and anxiety. It also offers antioxidant protection. Tuna, salmon, crimini and shitake mushrooms, asparagus, tomatoes, brown rice, sweet potato, green vegetables, cantaloupe and summer squash are but some of the foods containing niacin.

B5 is pantothenic acid and is known as the anti-aging vitamin. It is also required for cell processes and optimal maintenance of fat. Foods high in B5 include baker's yeast, liver, chicken, sunflower seeds, shitake mushrooms, avocados, meat, wheat germ and sun dried tomatoes.

B6 helps us resist disease, while B7 makes our nails, skin and hair healthy. B9 is folic acid and helps to synthesize and repair our DNA cells.

B12 is considered the most important of the B-complex vitamins. It is essential for the manufacture of red blood cells and a deficiency of this vitamin can cause many issues such as anemia and peripheral neuropathy, a debilitating condition. B12 is also important to nerve cell function and is required for the replication of DNA. When this vitamin is deficient, our DNA cannot replicate normally. This means we cannot generate new, healthy cells and will experience the effects of aging.

It is not as hard as you think to include the Complex B's into your daily diet. Try gluten-free spaghetti with grass-fed meat sauce and add onions, spinach and shitake mushrooms. The ingredients in this dish, which includes tomatoes, will help to replenish any deficiencies in your B-complex vitamin level. Said another way, gluten-free spaghetti and meatballs can keep you looking young!

Vitamin C and Beta-Carotene:

Vitamin C is a powerful, safe, effective and important antioxidant for the growth and repair of all tissues in the body. It offers protection against immune system deficiencies, strokes, cardiovascular disease, the common cold and more. It is also believed to be an important supplement for those with dementia.

German researchers from the University of Ulm with Epidemiologist Professor Gabriele Nagel and Neurologist Professor Christine von Arnim, discovered that the blood-concentration of the antioxidants vitamin C and beta-carotene are significantly lower in patients with mild dementia than in healthy individuals. This involved a small study of seventy-four Alzheimer's patients and 158 healthy people, ages sixty-five to ninety. Other factors could have influenced the findings, such as whether the participants smoked or drank alcohol.

Folic Acid:

There is much debate as to whether folic acid can improve cognitive issues. Many studies have been done, all with differentiating results.

A research team led by Dr. Jane Durga of Wageningen University and Wageningen Center for Food Sciences, the Netherlands, performed a trial called Folic Acid and Carotid Intima-media Thickness (FACIT). They examined the possible link between folic acid and hardening of the arteries in 818 men and women ages fifty to seventy. The participants, who at the start of the trial had low folic acid levels in their blood, were provided with either 800 micrograms of folic acid or a placebo every day for three years. They were tested on memory, movement speed, information processing speed, and word fluency. In the Lancet medical journal, the researchers reported that those participants given folic acid showed significantly better changes in cognitive skills.

Another study done in 2005 with researchers from Jack Hopkins University, Baltimore, revealed that homocysteine (a non-protein amino acid produced by the body) is elevated in the blood when a person's folic acid intake is too low. Researchers found a clear link between homocysteine levels and cognitive ability. The researchers concluded that higher homocysteine levels were associated with worse function across a broad range of cognitive domains, and that homocysteine may be a potentially important modifiable cause of cognitive dysfunction.

Magnesium:

Exciting preliminary research strongly suggests that an increase in magnesium levels in the brain decreases the symptoms of Alzheimer's.

This can be accomplished by eating foods rich in this mineral, such as kelp, almonds, cashews, molasses, brazil nuts, pecans, to name a few and supplementing the diet with added magnesium.

Magnesium is a truly lifesaving mineral and unfortunately as much as 80% of Americans are deficient in it. It is required for the production of all proteins, including those that interact with vitamins A and D.

This mineral is required for more than 300 biochemical reactions in the body. An optimum level of magnesium helps the body maintain normal muscle and nerve function, keeps heart rhythm steady, and supports the immune system. Sufficient magnesium in one's diet also improves sleep. The sleep hormone called melatonin is disturbed when the body is deficient in magnesium. Serotonin, which relaxes the nervous system and elevates mood, depends upon magnesium. It is required for the growth and strength of muscles and loosens tight muscles, giving the body more flexibility. In building bone strength, magnesium is one of the most essential minerals because it stimulates a hormone called calcitonin, which builds strength in bones. It also suppresses a hormone called parathyroid that breaks down bone.

The list of health benefits is ongoing. Magnesium alkalizes and hydrates the body with necessary electrolytes and helps to relieve constipation. This mineral is also required to make hundreds of enzymes work, all the while assisting thousands of others. Most importantly, Magnesium helps to facilitate sugar metabolism.

FAT SOLUBLE VITAMINS:

To comprehend fat-soluble vitamins, we must understand that vitamins A, D, and K work together and also with minerals like magnesium and zinc, with dietary fat, and with key metabolic factors like carbon dioxide and thyroid hormone. This is reason to exercise caution about optimal supplement dosages of these vitamins. Again I stress that you consult a physician on what fat-soluble supplements to take and suggested dosages.

Vitamin A, D and K2:

Vitamins A, D and K2 work synergistically to support immune health and strong bones and teeth and to protect soft tissues from calcification.

Vitamins A and D support the absorption of zinc, which supports the absorption of all fat-soluble vitamins.

Vitamin K activates proteins by adding carbon dioxide to them. We can increase carbon dioxide production by consuming carbohydrates, by exercising and by maintaining strong thyroid status.

Vitamin D is a fat-soluble hormone that helps regulate the immune system and helps the body absorb calcium and phosphorus, important elements for building and keeping bones strong. New research also shows that vitamin D may help to prevent obesity, several cancers, cardiovascular disease, autoimmune disorders, arthritis, psoriasis, diabetes, psychosis, and respiratory infections including colds and flu.

Vitamin D is important for the person with dementia. This vitamin has shown to improve a variety of brain disorders, including Alzheimer's. A new study reveals that vitamin D deficiency is associated with a substantial increased risk of dementia and Alzheimer's disease in older people.

Just published in Neurology and Science Daily, an international team led by Dr. David Llewellyn from the University of Exeter Medical School in the UK investigated the study's participants. The study consisted of 1,658 elderly American adults (aged sixty-five and over) who were initially free from dementia, cardiovascular disease, and stroke. The participants were then followed for six years to determine who developed Alzheimer's disease and other types of dementia. During the study, 171 participants developed all-cause dementia, including 102 cases of Alzheimer's disease.

The study also revealed that elderly Americans who were moderately deficient in vitamin D had a 53% increased risk of developing dementia of any kind. The risk increased to 125% in those who were severely deficient in this vitamin.

Difference between Vitamin D2 and Vitamin D3:

Most people think that if they are not getting enough vitamin D from the sun, they should consume foods fortified with vitamin D. Foods fortified with vitamin D contain D2 (calciferol), a plant-based form that comes from irradiated mushrooms and is considered by many doctors to be much less well utilized by the body than vitamin D3.

Vitamin D3 comes from three natural sources; exposure to sunlight, in foods like oily fish and through added pharmaceutical-grade supplements. The older we get the less efficient our body becomes at converting sunlight into vitamin D.

Hence a pharmaceutical-grade vitamin D supplement is important for elderly people, especially those with dementia.

Vitamin D3 (cholecalciferol) is an animal-based form made from sheep's wool, and is considered by most doctors to be the best form. It is the natural form that the body makes from sunlight.

On the advice of our physician, Jack and I take 2000 IU of D3 during the winter months in Canada when the sun is down south in Florida bathing and we are surviving in -20 degree Celsius weather conditions.

Coenzyme Q10:

Coenzyme Q10, also known as ubiquinone or coenzyme Q or CoQ10, is a fat-soluble vitamin essential for energy production in our cells. It is required to convert the energy from fats and sugars you eat into usable cellular energy. It is a fact that the body's natural production of CoQ10 declines significantly with age. Add to this that statin drugs deplete CoQ10 levels in the blood and tissues.

CoQ10 also helps the body neutralize harmful free radicals. This nutrient reduces our overall risk of developing chronic diseases. Our heart, kidney and liver possess the highest concentrations of this vitamin because these organs require the most energy to function.

Much controversy exists as to whether Coenzyme Q10 in supplement form can benefit brain health. So it's important to eat foods rich in CoQ10. Beef is the richest source of CoQ10. Some studies have shown that absorption of the ubiquinol form of CoQ10 is greater than the conventional ubiquinone form. But some doctors believe that the ubiquinone form is just as good. Be sure to seek advice by your physician on the best form for you.

The use of anticholinergic medications (used for gastrointestinal, respiratory and genitourinary disorders, insomnia, and dizziness), pain relievers, antihistamines, antidepressants, narcotic pain relievers, and statin-based cholesterol medications all deplete the brain of CoQ10 and neurotransmitter precursors. They prevent the delivery of essential fatty acids and fat-soluble antioxidants to the brain by inhibiting the production of low-density lipoprotein. For this reason these medications are believed by many experts to increase the risk of dementia.

Much controversy exists as to whether Coenzyme Q10 in supplement form can benefit brain health. Dr. Levy believes this product to be beneficial to the brain and in slowing the progression of dementia.

Note that water-soluble formulations of CoQ10 and ubiquinol have been developed which don't require fats or oils and can significantly increase the amounts of CoQ10 and ubiquinol in the bloodstream.

SUPPLEMENTS:

Omega 3 Fatty Acids:

Omega 3 essential fatty acids play an important role in the body and the structure of our brain cells. Their most crucial role is in the prevention of cardiovascular diseases like heart attacks and strokes.

Theoretically, we should get these fats through our daily diets. This is certainly not the case for most people; especially if you eat fish and beef but once per month. Hence we should rely upon an Omega 3 supplement.

There are three main fatty acids. They are:

- alpha-linolenic acid (ALA) from vegetable oils, nuts and seeds
- docosahexaenoic acid (DHA) from oily fish, such as salmon and mackerel
- eicosapentaenoic acid (EPA) from oily fish such as salmon and mackerel

Alpha-linolenic acid (ALA):

The body lacks the ability to make ALA naturally and so it is important to consume foods rich in this fatty acid. ALA provides the body with energy and is a primary building block for DHA and EPA. Vegetables, nuts and seeds are rich in ALA, with flaxseed believed to be the richest.
Some research suggests that a sufficient level of ALA can be converted to DHA and EPA. But this conversion is still unreliable. The reason is that the conversion requires a sufficient level and combination of B3, B6, vitamin C, zinc and magnesium. If the body is deficient in one or any of these vitamins and minerals the conversion fails. ALA is important to our health, to provide energy, support the other fatty acids DHA and EPA, to support many body systems, and to decrease the risk of chronic diseases.
There is growing research, studies and literature linking sufficient Omega 3 dietary consumption with brain function, with an emphasis on DHA and EPA.

Docosahexaenoic acid (DHA):

DHA makes up on average 15% to 20% of all fat in our brain. Drops in DHA brain levels are known to be associated with cognitive impairment. DHA is considered a valuable anti-inflammatory for the body and brain and is particularly important to brain function. It kick starts the growth of new neurons in the brain, leading to improved memory and the repairing of cognitive decline.

Eicosapentaenoic acid (EPA):

EPA contributes toward the proper function of our nervous system, including our brain and depends on the presence of DHA. Our risk of developing excessive inflammation and inflammation-related diseases can be lowered through consumption of foods rich in EPA. The only way to control cellular inflammation in the brain is to maintain high levels of EPA in the blood. A sufficient level of EPA is also important in the preventing and slowing of dementia.

Published in Neurology, a new study showed that an increased intake of Omega 3 fatty acids has been linked to a boost in later life brain volume, associated with brain health and warding off dementia.

Krill Oil:

Some people prefer to obtain their Omega 3's with Krill oil. Krill is the Norwegian word for 'whale food.' Its oil comes from a tiny, shrimp-like crustacean. Primarily whale sharks, mantas and Baleen whales eat this animal. They make up the largest animal biomass on the planet and are an essential building block in the marine food chain. They feed on plant matter and occur low in the ocean food chain, thus being free of heavy metals, PCB's and dioxins.

Krill oil contains fifty times more antioxidants than fish oil, thus preventing the highly perishable Omega 3 fats from oxidizing before you are able to absorb them into your cellular tissue. It is believed to combat ageing, heart disease, high cholesterol, high blood pressure, strokes, cancer, osteoarthritis, depression and Alzheimer's. Additionally, the Omega 3 in Krill is attached to phospholipids that increase its absorption. This means you need less of it, and it will not cause belching or burping like many other fish oil products.

Pyrroloquinoline Quinone (PQQ):

With age our mitochondria (the powerhouses of our cells) become damaged and weak and die off with age. PQQ is a potent antioxidant that triggers mitochondrial that activates the genes that give birth to new powerhouse generators in our cells. Brain cells need a lot of energy to be able to communicate with each other and to also communicate with the body. Muscle also needs a lot of energy to help us move. PQQ promotes cellular function in three ways. It activates genes that promote the formation of fresh mitochondria. It interacts with genes directly involved in

130

mitochondrial health, and it supports healthy body weight, normal fat and sugar metabolism.

Resveratrol:

In having made my living for over the past 2.5 decades as a wine writer, author and wine judge, I am familiar with the magical antioxidant called resveratrol. It possesses anti-oxidant, anti-inflammatory and anti-carcinogenic properties.

It is at the heart of the French Paradox, an idea that came to light in the 1980's. The French Paradox summarizes the paradoxical idea that French people who eat foods high in saturated fat and drink generous amount of wine, have a relatively low rate of coronary heart disease. This antioxidant can be found in red wine, grapes, chocolate and peanuts.

Vitamin E:

Oxidation is a natural process that takes place during normal cellular function. While the body metabolizes oxygen efficiently, about 1% to 2% of cells will get damaged during the process and turn into free radicals. Free radicals are damaged cells that can be problematic. They are called 'free' because these cells are void of a critical molecule. They are like vampires on a rampage to pair with another molecule. They kill cells to acquire their missing molecule and they injure the cells, thus damaging the DNA, creating the seed for disease. External toxins like air pollution, cigarette smoke, pesticides, excessive alcohol are examples of free-radical generators.

Our body simply does not produce enough antioxidants and so we need to ingest more fruits and vegetables and vitamin supplementations to get sufficient antioxidants to keep our body healthy.

Vitamin E is a fat-soluble antioxidant. In connection with vitamins A and C and Beta-carotene, it neutralizes the free-radical assault.

Vitamin E should not be taken in high dosage by all persons with Alzheimer's or dementia. As I stress, be sure to consult your physician before adding this vitamin or any vitamin to your regime.

In an organic nutshell:

a) Research shows that vitamin E supplementation can slow functional decline in those with Alzheimer's.
b) Vitamins are not created equal.
c) Take supplements made from organic whole food sources that are GMO free.
d) Choose liquid forms over tablets and capsules when possible.
e) Take pharmaceutical grade vitamins and supplements.
f) On vitamins and supplements look for an indication on the bottle that says 'this product is laboratory tested and its potency is guaranteed.'
g) Look for an expiration date.
h) If you have dementia or you are the caregiver of someone with dementia talk to your naturopathic doctor, physician or functional medicine physician about implementing the following vitamins and supplements into both of your daily regimes:
   - Vitamin B 1, 6 and 12 (sublingual)
   - Omega-D3 Liquid
   - Vitamin D3
   - Mito-Matrix Advanced Antioxidant
   - High Count, Multi-Strain Acidophilus and Bifidus
   - Cogni-Q (PQQ + CoQ10)
   - Vitamin E
   - Multi vitamin
   - Coconut oil or MCT oil (caprylic acid)
   - Curcumin (turmeric)

Chapter 13: Brain Foods and Spices

As much as we are dependent on supplements, they cannot fill the gap in our diet. Vitamins and supplements are not a substitute for the nutrients and benefits available through eating whole foods. Whole foods contain literally thousands of phytochemicals, fiber, nutrients and minerals that work together to help prevent deficiencies and disease and to promote over all good health. These elements cannot be substituted or duplicated with any vitamin-supplement cocktail.
Foods high in vitamins A, E, B, C, folic acid and magnesium have a positive impact on the brain and improve alertness and memory.

Almonds:

Nuts, specifically almonds, should be an integral part of your Dementia Diet for many reasons. They are a healthy fat that alkalizes the body, nourishes the nervous system and aids weight loss and helps to control weight. They are low glycemic and help lower the rise in blood sugar and insulin after meals. According to research conducted at Tufts University in Medford, Massachusetts, USA, the flavonoids in the skins of almonds work in harmony with vitamin E, reducing the risk of heart disease and protecting the artery walls from damage. In fact, consuming almonds five times per week reduces one's risk of a heart attack by 50%, according to the Loma Linda University School of Public Health in California. Most importantly, almonds contain riboflavin and L-carnitine that boost brain activity. Studies suggest that almonds can reduce the risk of Alzheimer's disease.

Blueberries:

Blueberries help to protect the brain from oxidative stress and may reduce the effects of Alzheimer's disease and dementia. Studies show that diets rich in blueberries can significantly improve the learning capacity and motor skills of aging rats, making them mentally equivalent to much younger rats.

Cashews, Hazelnuts, Peanuts and Pecans:

All these nuts are high in Omega 3 and Omega 6's, vitamin E, folate, vitamin B6 and magnesium – vitamins and minerals that are believed to help prevent and slow the progression of dementia.

Cinnamon:

Every morning my father puts cinnamon on a quarter slice of toast with peanut butter and eats it. Since undertaking this morning ritual, he says he no longer experiences angina when he walks. Cinnamon has many health benefits for the body and the brain, including anti-viral and anti-bacterial properties to help to heal irritable bowel syndrome, gastric cancers and stomach flus, as well as colds, a sore throat and cough.

It possesses two compounds called cinnamaldehyde and epicatechin that aid in preventing clumps of the tau protein from occurring in the brain, and therefore is believed to help prevent Alzheimer's. Cinnamon also regulates insulin levels for diabetics. And for this reason studies suggest that it may also contain anti-Alzheimer's properties.

Cruciferous Vegetables:

According to a paper co-authored by Samueli Institute Senior Fellow Harald Walach, Ph.D., and published in the Journal of Nutrition, Health and Aging in 2012, consuming at least three servings of cruciferous vegetables (broccoli, kale, cauliflower, Brussels sprout) each day can have a significant impact on lowering the risk of dementia and the rate of cognitive decline.

These vegetables possess folate and carotenoids that lower homo-cysteine, an amino acid linked to cognitive impairment.

Leafy Greens:

Kale, spinach, collard and mustard greens are examples of leafy greens. Leafy greens have concentrated levels of minerals,

134

phytonutrients and vitamins B, E, K and C, as well as beta-carotene, zeaxanthin and lutein. They are also rich in iron, magnesium, calcium and potassium. The top leafy greens include spinach, mustard greens, collards, Swiss chard and romaine lettuce. We eat leafy greens on a regular basis. I make an Asian-inspired vinaigrette combining a dash of sesame oil with equal parts rice vinegar and Kikkoman salt reduced soy sauce (gluten-free), sesame seeds and freshly grated ginger. These foods are rich in folate and B9, improving cognition and reducing depression.

Whole grains:

Chapter 5 covers a list of low-glycemic grains that are healthy for the body and the brain.

Pumpkin, squash, asparagus, tomatoes, and beets:

High in vitamin A, folate and iron, these vegetables, when steamed or not over-cooked support healthy cognition.

Seeds: Hemp, Pumpkin Seeds, Sesame Seeds, Sunflower Seeds:

Seeds are packed with vitamin B15. They improves circulation, lower blood cholesterol, support the immune system, and increase energy levels.

We don't usually hear a lot about vitamin B15. Also known as Pangamic Acid, vitamin B-15 is a controversial vitamin in North America. It has been removed from B-Complex supplements. The FDA took Pangamic Acid products off the market over twenty years ago. Other countries like Russia have been using this vitamin, believing it treats a variety of symptoms and diseases. It is used in this country (Canada) to treat alcoholism, drug addiction, aging and senility, autism, heart disease and more.

By enhancing liver function, Pangamic acid gently stimulates the endocrine and so acts as a detoxifier.

Because of its interactions with other vitamins, it's best to stick to eating foods that contain it rather than looking for a supplement.

Turmeric:

It is now a scientific fact that curcumin, an antioxidant compound found in the root of the turmeric plant, is one of the most powerful natural brain protecting substances in the world. We take turmeric everyday in the form of a supplement called 'highly bioavailable curcumin.' Jack and I also regularly visit a restaurant called House of India in our city. We love curry. Curcumin in turmeric is believed to prevent the spread of amyloid protein plaques that cause dementia. In Japan physicians at Kariya Toyota General Hospital in Kariya City evaluated three case studies involving turmeric and concluded that the herb showed relief of dementia symptoms and improved overall cognitive function. The study involved patients taking turmeric capsules for one year, which found improvements with their symptoms. (See my Dementia Diet Chai Latte Recipe in the book called Dementia Diet: Getting Started.)

In an organic nutshell:

Also incorporate into your diet:
- Low glycemic whole grains
- Nuts and seeds.
- Leafy greens
- Crucifer vegetables
- Blueberries
- Cinnamon
- Turmeric (curcumin)

The Author: About Shari Darling

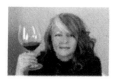

Shari Darling is the CEO of Understand Publishing
http://understandpublishing.com and also the CEO of
www.dementiadiet.net and www.dementiadietshop.com

As well as being a full time caregiver to her husband Jack, Shari is also an International award-winning and best-selling author and journalist, educator, TV and radio host and wine judge. She specializes in food, wine, cheese and Gluten-Free and the partnership between them.

Shari's concepts in sensory science as it pertains to wine and food pairing and her learning tools are utilized in colleges and universities throughout Canada for chef and sommelier training, including George Brown College, Niagara College and Brock University.

She has been the newspaper columnist for the Peterborough Examiner (Sunmedia) in Peterborough, Ontario, Canada for over a decade and writes for several other magazines. She is the creator of wine-related products and books which are celebrated under three series called Wine Pairing Club Presents; Cheesemaking; The Gluten-Free Club.

Shari and Jack are now focused on the Dementia Diet brand to fulfill their mission to impact the epidemic of dementia.

For More Information go to www.dementiadiet.net

THE END

Printed in Great Britain
by Amazon